Having Nasal Surgery?
Don't You Become An
Empty Nose Victim!

Christopher Martin, N.C.S.P.
Foreword by Steven M. Houser, M.D.,
Leading Medical Authority on Empty Nose Syndrome

Library of Congress Control Number: 2007934695

Having Nasal Surgery? Don't You Become An Empty Nose Victim!
is dedicated to empty nose syndrome patients who suffer,
often in silence, and feel depleted of hope, energy and life.

Disclaimer

⊶⊷

The information presented in this book is non-professional advice based upon my personal experiences as a nasal and sinus sufferer diagnosed with rhinosinusitis, allergic rhinitis and empty nose syndrome (ENS). As an empty nose sufferer and layperson, I do not have a medical degree or training. I am not a healthcare professional, but someone expressing my personal beliefs and sharing my subjective symptoms of ENS, along with what has worked for me in treating it. While these treatments have been effective for me, everyone responds differently to them so what helped me might not benefit someone else. I strongly recommend you discuss treatment ideas in this book with your doctor before attempting them. The best course of action with any health-related problem is consultation with a medical professional, and I take no responsibility for decisions made by people who read this book.

Further, the views and interpretations of the science of ENS, turbinate surgeries, politics of ENS, why ENS is difficult to diagnose, and discussion of postnasal drip represent lay opinion. The strength of this book is I, a layperson, personally suffer from ENS whereas most doctors do not and only treat it.

I also acknowledge that CT scan pictures in this book are not exact anatomic representations, but are for illustrative purposes. The first 3 case examples of ENS patients in chapter 1 are fictitious, although they are accurate representations of what many ENS sufferers experience.

The case examples in chapter 8 are also fictitious. Any similarity to individual persons, either living or dead, is coincidental.

Finally, I would like to protect the identities of ear, nose and throat (ENT) specialists who have treated me for nasal and sinus problems, including the doctor whose surgery resulted in ENS. Although I concede feeling frustration with ENT doctors who seem unaware of ENS symptoms, most have still been helpful in their respective ways and I am thankful for treatments they have provided. Therefore, I only identify ENT doctors who have been most helpful to me.

Table of Contents

Acknowledgments

First and foremost, I would like to thank my Savior and Lord Jesus Christ for giving me strength, endurance and compassion to write this book.

I would like to thank my beautiful wife, Colleen, who was supportive while I spent endless hours writing and thinking about this book. She is a source of great support and inspiration to me, during good times and bad. I also thank my daughters, Faith and Abigail, who are a great source of joy in my life along with our unborn baby who will be born around Christmas 2007.

I would like to show gratitude toward my father who drove with me to Cleveland, Ohio, where I underwent the Alloderm® implants. He accompanied me during these procedures and was very supportive. He also spent time reviewing the book and offering feedback.

I would like to thank other family members for their love and support, including my mother; my two sisters, Lori and Robin, and their families; my maternal grandmother; and my in-laws, the Kissel family; as well as family members not mentioned.

I have been overwhelmed by the outpouring of support from, and would like to express my deep thanks and gratitude to, the following doctors:

- Dr. Steven Houser of Cleveland, Ohio, an excellent ear, nose and throat (ENT) specialist who provided me with two implant operations (which have been beneficial). Dr. Houser is also a dedicated humanitarian to those suffering from empty nose syndrome (ENS) by providing a wealth of information for people with ENS, and examining numerous patients and voluntarily evaluating hundreds of computed tomography (CT) scans of ENS patients. Not only has Dr. Houser been generous enough to write the foreword for this book, but also his support, insights and encouragement gave me ambition to write it. You can visit his website at *www.geocities.com/shouser144/index.html*.

• Dr. Murray Grossan of Los Angeles, California, who developed the Hydro Pulse® Nasal-Sinus Irrigation System and wrote *The Sinus Cure* and *How to Be Free of Sinus Disease—Permanently!*, all of which has been tremendously helpful in my treatment of ENS. Dr. Grossan is a practicing ENT specialist at Cedars-Sinai Medical Center. He read this book and has offered much support and numerous helpful suggestions. You can visit his non-commercial website at *www.ent-consult.com*, and his commercial website at *www.hydromedonline.com*.

• Dr. Wellington Tichenor of New York, New York, who read this book and offered constructive feedback, and was generous enough to write the introduction for this book. Dr. Tichenor is a medical specialist in sinusitis who does not perform surgery, but primarily treats patients who have not responded well to surgery, such as ENS patients. Dr. Tichenor is a leader in both prevention and treatment of ENS. His website, *www.sinuses.com*, has won numerous awards for outstanding content.

• Dr. Eugene Kern of Rochester, Minnesota, who read this book and offered positive, constructive feedback. Dr. Kern is a practicing ENT specialist at the Mayo Clinic, and former president of the American Rhinologic Society from 1981-1982 and of the

International Rhinologic Society from 1996-2000. Dr. Kern coined the term "empty nose syndrome" in 1994. After treating patients with ENS for many years, he gave a series of lectures on this topic and later summarized his findings in a research article, "Atrophic Rhinitis: A Review of 242 Cases."

- Other doctors who have provided me with care as I have struggled to treat my nose.

I would like to further express appreciation for the help of friends including, but not limited to:

- Ben Hower, who spent numerous hours reviewing and editing this book and offered helpful suggestions to greatly enhance the final product.
- Vincent Rondenelli, who drew 7 pictorial drawings for this book.
- Amanda Butler, the senior designer at Cold Tree Press who worked on and corresponded with me regarding numerous details of this book, from designing the cover to formatting the interior. Her expertise and dedication significantly enhanced the finished product.
- Margy Olmstead, an expert indexer from Oak Grove Indexing Services at *www.oakgroveindex.com*, who created a fine index for this book.
- Other friends not mentioned.

Foreword

By Dr. Steven M. Houser

I first encountered empty nose syndrome (ENS) during my fourth year of residency. I assisted Dr. X in nasal surgery that included septoplasties and turbinate reductions. I witnessed Dr. X take angled nasal scissors, press the cutting surface against the front of the inferior turbinate, cut and push the mucosa off the inferior turbinate, and finally withdraw a lengthy segment of mucosal tissue that looked like a long slug. I pulled packs from these patients' noses the day after surgery and always prayed their bleeding would stop and I would not need to repack them.

Several months into the rotation I was in clinic with Dr. X. I picked up a chart to see the next patient who presented with nasal issues. I went into the room and introduced myself to a middle-aged African American woman. She complained of nasal blockage and congestion, and her breathing seemed problematic. Dr. X operated on her nose several years prior and she was no better now; in fact, she seemed worse. Interestingly, she mentioned that she seemed to breathe better with a cold. Then I examined her and was shocked to see an enormous airway. I could see her soft palate with ease, as the inferior turbinates were just a small ridge on each side.

Why did this woman complain of poor breathing with such an open nose? I was baffled. I presented the case to Dr. X who hemmed and hawed and was unable to explain the symptoms either.

From that point forward I set out to answer why this might be and came in contact with Dr. Murray Grossan; we became fast friends. I began to think about ENS, and I researched the topic as thoroughly as possible. Eventually I decided to begin reconstructing these patients by simulating their missing turbinates. I would like to think that I have made some patients feel better over the years through understanding and explanation, as well as surgical implantation.

Chris came to me after I had been doing ENS repairs for a while. He was missing significant tissue and, after doing a cotton test, I sized an appropriate implant that has resulted in improvement of his ENS symptoms. He later underwent a second implant surgery in February 2007, which has offered further benefit.

Chris' story is a compelling one. He tells a very personal tale to help inspire others. Chris also explores the science behind ENS to really inform others with similar difficulties. His advice to ENS patients is right on target. I hope this book will get the attention it deserves. I will certainly recommend it to the ENS patients I treat.

Dr. Houser is an ENT specialist at MetroHealth Medical Center and the Cleveland Nasal, Sinus and Sleep Center. He is also an assistant professor of Otolaryngology-Head and Neck Surgery at Case Western Reserve University.

Introduction

By Dr. Wellington S. Tichenor

I became interested in empty nose syndrome (ENS) when I started treating a large number of sinusitis patients 20 years ago.

I have been overwhelmed by the devastation that ENS patients experience. As a result of an iatrogenic (caused by medical treatment) origin, the lives of these productive individuals have been profoundly affected. Before their surgery they could go about their lives with varying degrees of difficulty, but after it they were completely disabled.

I recall one patient who was the president of a large corporation. He had to retire precipitously because of his inability to continue in the high degree of responsibility. This patient became so focused on the debilitation caused by ENS that it became hard for him to do anything else. He described himself as a quadruple amputee (the middle and inferior turbinates were removed on both sides). He even wrote a poem entitled "Ode to the Turbinates."

As a medical specialist in sinusitis, I primarily treat patients who previously had unsuccessful surgery. Many of them consequently suffer from both sinusitis and ENS. As a result of my website, *Sinusitis: A Treatment Plan that works for Allergy and Asthma too* at *www.sinuses.com*, I receive a large number of emails from those who have previously had surgery, but have not improved. Like my own patients, many of these emails are from ENS sufferers.

Yet it is important to point out that some patients who have extensive turbinate surgery do not appear to suffer—the lucky ones who manage not to have such severe symptoms despite extensive tissue loss. Unfortunately, we figure out afterwards which patients can safely have more tissue removed versus those who will be more devastated. Even so, it is also important to recognize that if patients don't have ENS as a result of turbinate surgery, they may still have recurrent sinusitis as a result of scar tissue formation.

Too many surgeons today believe they can indiscriminately remove large amounts of turbinate tissue and, indeed, there remains controversy in the field whether this surgery can be done with minimal complications. I am a strong proponent of conservative turbinate surgery that consists of removing the smallest amount of tissue possible.

Finally, there are very few of us physicians who know how to treat ENS patients. I hope this book can help ENS patients and those who may be able to avoid this terrible complication of surgery by directing them toward a treatment plan that works—not makes them worse!

Dr. Tichenor is a medical specialist in sinusitis in New York City. He also teaches a course on endoscopy in patients who previously underwent sinus surgery at the American Academy of Allergy, Asthma, and Immunology each year. Dr. Tichenor recently wrote a paper, "Nasal and Sinus Endoscopy for Medical Management of Resistant Rhinosinusitis, Including Postsurgical Patients," which will be published in the Journal of Allergy and Clinical Immunology *and is now available on the American Academy of Allergy, Asthma and Immunology website at www.aaaai.org.*

On a personal note, Dr. Tichenor is a chronic sinusitis sufferer who has had surgery twice, but was fortunate not to have much turbinate tissue removed. The surgeon only removed minimal turbinate tissue to access the sinuses he needed to operate on.

Having Nasal Surgery?

Don't You Become An

Empty Nose Victim!

———⊷⊷⊷———

Christopher Martin, N.C.S.P.

Chapter One

Empty Nose Syndrome

In spring 2003, a grateful lady traveled 75 miles to personally thank Dr. Murray Grossan of Los Angeles, California, a well-known ear, nose and throat (ENT)[a] specialist.[1] The reason: her son, then age 12, was scheduled for a bilateral turbinectomy, a surgery where inner nasal tissue known as turbinates is removed. But she read a 2001 *Los Angeles Times* article, "Sniffing at Empty Nose Idea" by Aaron Zitner, in which Dr. Grossan was cited as opposing such procedures because of potential complications such as ENS. Consequently, she cancelled the surgery, visited an allergist, and her son's nasal problems cleared. He was spared from becoming an ENS patient for life.

Others, however, are not so fortunate. They learn through personal experience that ENS means:

- Constant, panicky feeling of shortness of breath (despite a wide open nose).
- Chronic nasal dryness.
- Thick, sticky mucus.
- Diminished sense of smell.
- Disturbed sleep.
- Intolerance to cold, dry air.

---

a The terms ENT specialist, ENT doctor, ENT physician, and ENT surgeon are used interchangeably throughout the book to denote someone who is both a practicing doctor, some of whom also perform surgery. These professionals are the same as an otolaryngologist, although plastic surgeons also perform turbinate surgeries. Plastic surgeons and ENTs can work to prevent ENS as a complication of turbinate surgery and raise awareness of ENS. Since ENTs specialize in treating the nose, however, they are in a prime position to directly confront, diagnose, and remediate ENS sufferers.

- Anger, anxiety and depression.
- Disbelief from doctors at these symptoms.

Three case examples that demonstrate how ENS can adversely impact a patient's quality of life are as follows:

- "Elsie" was a popular girl who attended college for nursing and hoped to meet Mr. Right. After a turbinectomy she constantly felt fatigued, dropped out of college, her relationships with young men went downhill, and no medicine seemed to help. Most doctors did not seem to understand what she was going through, prescribing her medication for anxiety and depression. She has ENS.

- Before surgery, "Jim" seemed good-natured, confident, and ready to tackle most of life's challenges. Jim experienced mild sinus problems and had a deviated septum (crooked midline of the nose). He underwent a surgical procedure known as a septoplasty to straighten it, only to learn later that turbinate tissue was removed as well. After surgery, Jim felt dazed as though not enough oxygen reached his brain, and he rarely woke up feeling refreshed after a long night of sleep. He put cotton in his nose—anything to alleviate the dryness. Some doctors told him to "get over it" while others confirmed what he already suspected: he has ENS.

- Before surgery, "Mike" was full of energy. He enjoyed playing tennis and running, and could do either for 5 hours non-stop. After a turbinate surgery, he could neither run nor had much energy to play tennis, let alone for his job. Mike incurred severe breathing difficulties leading to significant difficulty concentrating, and recurrent sinus infections. Some doctors prescribed antibiotics, while one suggested even *more* removal of his turbinates. He has ENS.

Brief Background of Empty Nose Syndrome

ENS is a serious, iatrogenic medical condition that results from an ENT doctor or plastic surgeon removing too much turbinate tissue. Dr. Eugene Kern of the Mayo Clinic coined "empty nose syndrome" in summer 1994. Dr. Kern showed computed tomography (CT) scans of turbinate surgery patients to a visiting Swedish surgeon, Dr. Monica Stenquist. He suggested these scans indicated there was nothing in the nose and Dr. Stenquist replied they looked "empty," hence the term empty nose syndrome.[2]

The turbinates perform a number of important functions including directing airflow that enters the nose in a laminar (orderly) pattern, while also heating, humidifying, and filtering air. These functions help prepare air before it reaches the lungs. The turbinates also offer about 50% of nasal airflow resistance to the lungs, which is critical for optimal lung functioning. When too much turbinate tissue is removed, the nose is unable to perform these vital functions.

ENT doctors and plastic surgeons sometimes remove turbinate tissue after other interventions have been tried—including nasal steroid sprays, antihistamines, allergy shots, and decongestants—in attempt to make breathing easier by decreasing the size of enlarged turbinates that are blocking much of the nasal airway. (This enlargement is most often caused by allergic rhinitis, vasomotor rhinitis (non-allergic rhinitis), overuse of intranasal decongestants, or it may be caused by a septal deviation.) While a conservative turbinate surgery can be beneficial in relieving symptoms associated with an enlarged turbinate such as stuffiness and headaches, a turbinate surgery resulting in ENS can be devastating.

A perplexing symptom of ENS is the sensation of a shortness of air or as though one cannot breathe adequately despite the nasal cavity being wide open, a phenomenon called paradoxical obstruction. Other symptoms include a chronically dry nose, difficulty concentrating, shallow sleep, frequent headaches, increased pulmonary reactivity to volatile compounds or airborne irritants, a diminished sense of smell, thick, sticky mucus, occasional crusting (dried mucus), occasional nosebleeds, sometimes recurrent sinus infections, and fatigue, all of which might lead to anxiety and depression.

"Severely debilitating," "horrible," "totally disabling," "troubling," "distressing," and leaving a patient feeling "miserable" are some ways prominent doctors have described ENS.[3-7] A high rate of ENS sufferers are anxious or depressed, and many are very preoccupied by their breathing difficulties.[8] Unlike temporary problems like a broken leg, breathing is constant and nasal breathing, which is far more satisfying and more protective against infection than mouth breathing, has been damaged.

Compare ENS with the following breathing disorders:

+ A chronic obstructive pulmonary disease (COPD) sufferer cannot get enough oxygen because of damage to his lungs. But at least with the oxygen tank he feels better.

+ A severe asthmatic suffers from less air to his lungs during an attack, but prescription medication or environmental changes help him feel better and he can return to a regular life.

Now imagine a condition where for 24-7 he feels like he is not getting enough air and neither oxygen nor medication helps improve his breathing difficulties. Worse yet, the doctors ignore him because his nose is "wide open." That is ENS.

The incidence of ENS is unknown, but it is possible there are millions of ENS sufferers in the United States with varying degrees of symptoms. These sufferers, who come from all walks of life, might not appropriately identify it or know what to do about it, while others might be going under the knife presuming they will enjoy nasal symptom improvement only to learn after surgery the operation left them with a more devastating problem: ENS.

Relationship between Sinusitis, Allergic Rhinitis, Asthma and ENS

It is important to first understand mucociliary clearance (MCC) to better understand how sinusitis, allergic rhinitis, asthma and ENS are interrelated. Like *many* ENS sufferers, I have allergic rhinitis because allergies often lead to enlarged turbinates, which doctors resect. Like *some* ENS sufferers, I have sinusitis because sinus surgery (for sinusitis) is sometimes performed in conjunction with turbinate surgery, the latter of which can cause ENS.

Mucociliary Clearance (MCC)

Mucous membranes (mucosa for short) are rich in glands that secrete mucus[b]. They line the nose, sinus cavities, respiratory and digestive tracts. Mucous membrane glands secrete between 1-2 liters of mucus per day. Mucus acts as the nose's first line of defense, providing surface area to trap foreign particles while also humidifying air.

Healthy ciliated cells beat at a rapid rate of 16 pulses per second and help move the mucus blanket along the mucous membrane to the throat,

---

b *The terms mucus and mucous are often confused. Mucus consists of 2 layers: the sol (thin) and gel (thick) layer above it. The gel layer traps particles and the entire mucus blanket—sol, gel, and particles—is transported per cilia to the pharynx (throat), where it is swallowed. Mucous membranes are rich in glands that produce mucus and are thus covered with mucus.*

esophagus and stomach. Stomach acid kills the bacteria, viruses, molds or fungi, the mucus is broken up, and it is ultimately excreted.

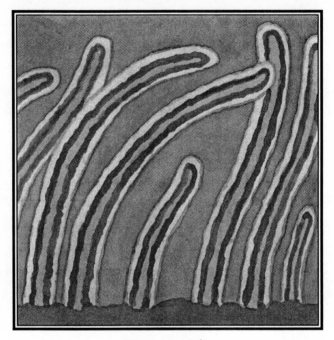

Figure 1. Cilia

When functioning properly, MCC happens without our notice. During times of mucosal inflammation, however, the mucous glands secrete even more mucus to fight off infections. The cilia slow down and mucus does not drain properly. For example, one study demonstrated nasal cilia of people with chronic sinusitis and postnasal drip beat at 6 pulses per second, which is much slower than the healthy cilia rate.[9] Consequently, stagnant mucus remains, bacteria multiply, and infection takes hold. Ultimately, long-term decreased mucociliary flow can make someone at increased risk for sinusitis and even lower respiratory problems such as asthma.

Basic Definitions of Inflammatory Disorders

1) *Allergic rhinitis* occurs because allergens (e.g., pollen, dust, mold, smoke) in the air cause an immune system response consisting of production of specific immunoglobin E (IgE); futher exposure leads to inflammation of the nasal membranes. IgE is an antibody (protein used by the immune system to fight infection). Symptoms including nasal congestion, clear nasal discharge, sneezing, nose and eye itching, and tearing eyes. Untreated allergies can over time lead to diminished nasal cilia functioning which, in turn, can predispose one to recurrent infections and sinusitis, which might partly explain why up to 80% of those with sinusitis also have allergies.[10]

2) *Sinusitis* is inflammation of the sinuses. The nose is considered the guardian of the lungs, so untreated sinusitis can lead to a weakened defense system and thereby exacerbate asthma symptoms. Not surprisingly, then, more than 50% of asthmatics have also suffered from chronic sinusitis at some point; and 15-56% of those with sinusitis or allergic rhinitis also have asthma.[11]

3) *Rhinosinusitis* is a newer term meaning inflammation of both the nose and sinuses. This term is used synonymously with and might be more accurate than sinusitis because, while it is possible to suffer from either inflammation of the nose (rhinitis) or sinuses (sinusitis) separately, most patients with inflammation of the sinuses also suffer from nasal inflammation. This is due to the interrelationship between the nose and sinuses. These terms are used interchangeably throughout this book.

4) *Asthma* is reversible constriction of the airways, which become inflamed and lined with excessive amounts of mucus. Symptoms include wheezing and shortness of breath. It follows, then, that ENS sufferers who also have asthma suffer from greater breathing difficulties than those with ENS alone.

Interestingly, 60% of asthma sufferers have allergy-induced asthma, which is when allergies trigger or cause asthma symptoms. So effectively treating allergies by following treatment strategies in this book can prevent or significantly improve asthma in many cases. Yet it is important to note an asthma sufferer must follow his or her doctor's orders and might need treatments specific to asthma, such as an inhaler, as well.

Dr. Terence Davidson of San Diego, California, who introduced the concept of adding antibiotics to pulsatile saline irrigation, posted the following hypothetical doctor-patient exchange on his website regarding consultation for allergy treatment, during which the patient inquired into surgical treatments for allergic rhinitis:[12]

Patient: I have heard that there are laser surgeries which at least reduce the symptoms of allergic rhinitis.

Doctor: Yes, there are all sorts of procedures using knives, cauteries, lasers, cold instruments, hot instruments, etc. All of these procedures are aimed at reducing the turbinates which are responsible for humidification, filtering and warming inspired air. If you damage enough of the turbinate, then your nose will remain open and the symptoms of the allergic rhinitis may be reduced.

Patient: That sounds like a good treatment to me. It certainly beats filling my body with steroids and twice daily controlled drownings *[referring to saline irrigation, which is an irrational fear as it does not happen with this technique]*.

Doctor: Well, while I appreciate your humor, there is a down side risk to turbinate surgery. Assuming the surgery goes well, the less invasive surgeries only work for a short period of time like a year, and then require repeat treatments. The more permanent procedures, like the laser surgery that you mentioned, leave your nose permanently damaged. Later in life when your mucosa undergoes a certain atrophy associated with aging, all of a sudden you do not have enough mucosa to maintain a humidified, filtered, and warmed inspiration, and your nose will become dry, crusty, infected and painful. This is a horrible condition. It is called atrophic rhinitis, or in some cases it is called *empty nose syndrome.*

My Own Approach to ENS

ENS is difficult to cope with and the subjective symptoms I constantly experience are painfully clear to me. Management of this condition is intense as it often consumes at least one hour of my day, every day, between saline rinses, preparation of tea and medicines, and environmental modifications. The bottom line is this: I know what I feel, and perception is reality for me and numerous other ENS sufferers. But I will not complain.

Regrettably, the doctor who performed my partial turbinectomy has since passed away. I hold no grudges against him. I forgive him. I have never felt anger toward him, only peace. Such anger serves little purpose and would be detrimental to myself, as it could "eat away at me." Besides, anger cannot reverse what happened.

My energy is thus best channeled in a positive direction, toward helping myself and others. Striving to treat ENS without complaint, holding no grudges toward anyone, and providing useful information on ENS to fellow sufferers are my goals.

Plight of the ENS Sufferer

Many ENS sufferers are angry at themselves for undergoing an overly aggressive turbinate surgery or their doctor for performing it, stating they would do anything to have their turbinates back. Some feel their quality of life has been severely compromised; some feel alone and misunderstood in their suffering; others seek frequent medical opinion in the hope that something, anything, can be done to alleviate their symptoms.

Doctors will often refer the ENS sufferer to a psychiatrist or mental health counselor because of depression. While counseling or psychotropic medication might be necessary, it does not solve the physical problem that might underlie the depression: ENS.

Most ENS sufferers claim they were not properly informed of the possible complication of ENS prior to undergoing an operation on their turbinates, and they question if the ENT doctor or plastic surgeon removed more tissue than they thought would be removed, which is consistent with my own experiences. Unfortunately, it is likely these doctors did not inform the patient of a possible ENS complication not only because mention of ENS might obviously confuse and frighten the patient, or reflect negatively on the doctor, but also because too many of these doctors appear to have poor understanding of ENS.[13]

This lack of awareness to a disease of nasal origin, such as ENS, has its roots. Dr. Maurice Cottle, founder of the American Rhinologic Society in 1954 and International Rhinologic Society in 1965, and advocate of submucosal implant surgeries for people with primary atrophic rhinitis, frequently claimed he observed symptoms stemming from a nasal origin that were, at times, not believed by doctors or even patients.[14]

Regrettably, current lack of doctor awareness of ENS has increased sufferer distress. Doctors are puzzled when they see a wide open nose but the patient reports he or she cannot breathe. They might downplay the symptoms or even blame the patient in these instances. Consequently, ENS patients are satisfied (often overly appreciative) to find a physician who understands ENS symptoms, let alone one who offers to treat it surgically. These physicians appear to represent a small minority.

No doubt ENT doctors have sympathy and want to help and offer practical suggestions for treating nasal problems. But when it comes to ENS it seems many are unsure how to help, neglecting to acknowledge subjective symptoms ENS sufferers experience on a daily basis. At least that has been my experience after visiting more than 15 ENT doctors during the past 10 years. After all, most of these doctors have never personally experienced ENS symptoms and they cannot learn about ENS from a textbook because, unlike atrophic rhinitis that has received much research attention over the past 100 years, this particular syndrome has received minimal research attention to date.

For now, people will continue to receive turbinate reduction procedures with varying degrees of success or failure. Regrettably, some will conclude the "real trouble" for them began after removal of too much turbinate tissue.

Who is this Book Written For?

A. ENS sufferers, along with their families and friends.

B. Anyone considering turbinate surgery.

C. ENT doctors, plastic surgeons, and scientists studying regenerative medicine.

D. Sinus, allergy and postnasal drip sufferers.

Rationale

Four Reasons for this Book

1. Raise awareness by demystifying ENS through reflections on my own experiences, along with a review of medical research.
2. Offer what I (and others) have found most beneficial for treating ENS symptoms.
3. Use this discussion as a starting point and direction for future research.
4. Provide encouragement and hope.

The first objective of this book is to offer an inside look into the world of ENS. The reader can learn about real symptoms I have experienced (and continue to experience) as an ENS sufferer and the response of ENT specialists who have treated me. My story could be useful as a starting point of discussion for ENS sufferers, as well as family, friends and others who are interested in learning about ENS so they too can better understand and help people dealing with ENS.

I also discuss the politics of ENS and why diagnosis is difficult to provide necessary context for the reader (and to document history of ENS). Many readers will wonder why ENT doctors and plastic surgeons have not properly addressed, diagnosed or treated ENS, and why some nasal surgeries[c] today still result in ENS; such discussions answer these questions.

---

c Nasal surgery refers to surgery of the turbinates or septum, while sinus surgery is surgery of the sinuses that is generally performed to either remove inflamed tissue or enable better drainage of mucus by creating artificial passageways. Therefore, only turbinate (not sinus) surgery can lead to ENS, unless surgery of the turbinates (especially the middle turbinate) was performed in conjunction with the sinus operation.

I further explain the science behind ENS symptoms. The reader can gain understanding of the anatomical and physiological basis of ENS symptoms. The science proves authenticity of this syndrome.

Next, I discuss turbinate surgeries to empower those who might be considering nasal surgery to understand which turbinate surgeries are more or less likely to lead to ENS. Patients can use this knowledge to make wise choices when discussing surgical options with their doctors.

The second objective is to share what I have found most helpful in treating ENS with the hope that others struggling with ENS would similarly benefit. Many proposed treatments for ENS are also beneficial for treating sinus and allergy problems, and in preventing the need for surgery that could lead to ENS. The treatment options presented are based on my experiences as an ENS sufferer. Recommending a wide range of non-surgical treatments, the emphasis is more on natural treatments (such as saline irrigation) since I have found them most beneficial. I discuss medications, which are an essential component for me in treating ENS, but I refer readers who wish to learn more about medications to other sources of information, such as their doctors or other sinus books.

The third objective is to foster awareness of ENS among doctors and scientists. These doctors can read a testimonial of someone who has experienced the debilitating effects of ENS. My hope is that ENT doctors and plastic surgeons would ensure a turbinate surgery does not result in ENS, and serve ENS sufferers better through improved diagnoses and more promising treatments.

Further, a scientist can have his or her interest piqued about ENS, so that he or she works harder to find a cure. A scientist studying regenerative medicine, for example, could actively seek to create turbinate tissue that might ultimately represent a cure for ENS.

I gratefully acknowledge that ENT doctors in recent years have begun to address ENS in peer-reviewed research. Two examples are the landmark study "Atrophic Rhinitis: A Review of 242 Cases" by Drs. Eric Moore and Eugene Kern, and "Empty Nose Syndrome Associated with Middle Turbinate Resection" by Dr. Steven Houser. Hopefully ENT doctors and plastic surgeons will become increasingly aware of ENS through these publications.

The fourth objective is to provide inspiration and hope to the injured patient. A severely injured ENS sufferer may not fully overcome the breathing difficulties, but his or her condition can improve to an extent through proper treatment, in turn lessening the stress associated with ENS.

Chapter 1 References

1. Grossan, M. (personal communication, January 10, 2007).

2. Zitner, A. (2001, May 10). Sniffing at Empty Nose Idea. *Los Angeles Times.*

3. Lisa Etkin v. Merk & Company, Inc. and Metropolitan Life Insurance Company (2001). No. 00-5467. The United States District Court for the Eastern District of Pennsylvania. [P. 3].

4. Houser, S.M. (2006a). *Frequently Asked Questions.* Retrieved November 24, 2006, from Rhinology/Allergy Pages Web site: *www.geocities.com/shouser144/ens5.html.* [Para. 3].

5. Davidson, T. (2003). *Consultation for Allergic Rhinitis.* Retrieved August 8, 2006 from Head and Neck Surgery Consultations Web site: *www.surgery.ucsd.edu/ent/ davidson/consult_allergic_rhinitis.html.* [Para. 78].

6. Metson, R., & Mardon, S. (2005). *The Harvard Medical Guide to Healing Your Sinuses.* New York, NY: McGraw-Hill. [P. 162].

7. Grossan, M. (2005). *Asthma and Sinusitis.* Retrieved November 24, 2006, from emedicine from webmd Web site: *www.emedicine.com/ent/topic516.htm.* [Section 9 of 11].

8. Tichenor, W.S. (2004). *The Empty Nose Syndrome.* Retrieved November 24, 2006, from the Persistent Sinusitis Despite Surgery Web site: *www.sinuses.com/postsurg.htm.*

9. Bleeker, J.D., & Hoeksema, P.E. (1971). A simple method of measure the ciliary beat rate of respiratory epithelium. *Acta Oto-Laryngologica,* 71, 426-429.

10. Bruce, D.F., & Grossan, M. (2001). *The Sinus Cure: 7 Simple Steps to Relieve Sinusitis and other Ear, Nose, and Throat Conditions.* New York: Ballantine Books. [P. 29].

11. Bruce & Grossan, 2001, P. 45.

12. Davidson, T. (2003). Consultation for Allergic Rhinitis. Retrieved August 8, 2006 from Head and Neck Surgery Consultations Web site: *www.surgery.ucsd.edu/ent/ davidson/consult_allergic_rhinitis.html.* [Paras. 75-78].

13. Houser, S.M. (2004, September). *Empty Nose Syndrome Associated with Middle Turbinate Resection.* Poster Presented at the meeting of the American Rhinologic Society, New York.

14. Timmons, B.H. & Ley, R., Eds. (1994). *Behavioral and Psychological Approaches to Breathing Disorders.* New York: Plenum Press.

Chapter Two

My Story: Prior to the Partial Turbinectomy

xperiencing ENS, it is difficult to fathom I was the picture of perfect health for most of my childhood and adolescent years. I had neither allergies nor sinus infections, and I breathed comfortably. I was rarely absent from school. Beginning in eighth grade I participated on the high school tennis team with unmitigated passion for the sport. A friend and I played for hours on end during evenings and weekends. In tenth grade I ran endless miles on the cross country team, or so it seemed. Occasionally, the cross country team would run 10 miles during a practice and I could do it with remarkable ease, although still fatigued by the end. In retrospect, it is hard for me to imagine all that after coming down with the pernicious condition of ENS.

A Deteriorating Nasal Health

My nasal health slowly, but insidiously deteriorated during my eleventh and twelfth grade years (1996-1997). I cannot pinpoint the cause for this decline as it did not occur all at once, and I am unaware of any behavior I engaged in that might have contributed to this spiraling decline, except for perhaps social stress associated with adolescent life. Nevertheless, I had contracted many sinus infections that often resulted in oral antibiotic treatment. My father and I took many trips to a hospital one hour away for medical opinion. It seemed all the antibiotics in the world did not help. I was clueless as to why my nose began giving me so many problems. It seemed something was wrong and I wanted a solution.

The 'Quick Fix' but a Lifetime of Regret

In spring 1997, after numerous visits to the hospital, we met with an ENT doctor who recommended I receive a combined septoplasty and partial turbinectomy. Those terms meant little to me then, but I am all too aware of their meanings today. The purpose of a septoplasty is to straighten a deviated septum. The purpose of a partial turbinectomy is to reduce by roughly two-thirds the size of the turbinates, which had become swollen and were obstructing my breathing to some extent. The doctor reasoned that by reducing the size of the turbinates I would be able to breathe more comfortably and ward off bacterial infections.

What was not explained to me was that allergies could have been a contributing factor to my enlarged turbinates, nor were other alternatives suggested. He could have suggested using more conservative, mucosa-sparing turbinate surgeries such as radiofrequency or outfracture, two surgeries that are discussed in chapter 5. Also not discussed with me were possible complications resulting from this surgery, such as ENS.

A few years prior to this surgery I had my wisdom teeth extracted. That surgery was a positive experience as I recall waking up throughout the day to delicious milkshakes provided by my mother, and I incurred few complications. I anticipated another surgery with good results, or at least I thought. This nasal surgery then seemed to be in my best inter-est, a light at the end of a tunnel. In retrospect, this surgery changed my life—for the worse. Little did I know I was just entering a tunnel.

Shortly After the Partial Turbinectomy

I recall awakening from this surgery with uncomfortable packing in my nose. Although many surgeries do not require packing, patients under-going surgery that does require packing would attest it makes a patient feel miserable and I recall feeling groggy, but that was just the *beginning*.

This was an inpatient surgery and the doctor removed the packing one day following it. I remember him informing me that removing the packing would be tantamount to being hit in the forehead with a hockey puck. That analogy was accurate because I recall blood streaming from my nose at breakneck speed when he removed them. I felt awful. It felt as though the doctor stood on my chest and yanked the packing with all his might. Again, that was just the *beginning*.

I recall my nasal passages feeling hot, dry and uncomfortable weeks after this surgery. I remember feeling a burning sensation through my nose and I felt dizzy. A huge amount of air could enter my nose, but breathing neither felt natural nor adequate.

I did not realize how dire the consequences were at this point, as I did not know what hit me. It was an uncomfortable feeling and to this day I have a hard time describing it. It felt as though my nose had stale blood in it, and I would frequently have difficulty blowing it. I still felt congested with significant nasal breathing difficulties, finding only occasional relief when blowing out thick mucus that was reluctant to exit my nose.

About one month after surgery I moved from the relatively humid climate (at least during the summer) of Upstate New York to the dry climate of Kansas for my first semester of college. It was during this time my nose seemed to worsen.

Breathing through my nose felt awkward and uncomfortable. Thick mucus was often trapped in my nose and blocked my breathing, which made breathing uncomfortable and often uneven between nostrils. My thoughts were preoccupied with my nose as I frequently strained to simply breathe correctly. Finally, when I mustered enough strength to blow out mucus, it came in large chunks. The mucus felt hard and sometimes was unusually big, perhaps the size of a gumball.

Follow-up care for my nose was insufficient. I only had two follow-up visits with the ENT doctor in New York who performed the surgery. Each office visit he removed large bits of mucus, providing temporary nasal relief. I knew something seemed wrong with my nasal condition, but the ENT doctor did not appear concerned. His nonchalant demeanor regarding my condition during the weeks following surgery was an indication he likely believed this surgery represented success. Yet his analysis of my nasal health was incorrect because I physically felt more awful than ever and could not understand why. I trusted, or at least hoped, my condition would improve over time. I could not have been more wrong.

I tried not to complain, but sometimes it was hard not to. When I complained about my worsened nasal condition after the partial turbinectomy, I recall someone reminding me how I had nasal problems prior to the surgery. While this statement did not do justice to what I was feeling after surgery, it was accurate. I incurred frequent nasal infections prior to my partial turbinectomy and I rue that medical interventions, such as allergy medicine or saline irrigation, were not attempted prior to undergoing surgery. Like many ENS sufferers, I think "if only I knew then what I know now," because symptoms after surgery were certainly worse than the ones before it.

These symptoms included:
+ Chronic shortness of breath, which led to difficulty concentrating.
+ Chronic dryness.
+ Irritated mucous membranes, usually including an irritated throat (due to dryness).
+ Thick, sticky mucus.
+ Blood-tinged mucus.

Interestingly, one study suggested that harmful changes to nasal membranes resulting from a total inferior turbinectomy can actually lead to chronic sinusitis. [d,1] In that study some people who did not have chronic sinusitis *before* the turbinectomy developed it *after* the surgery.

I Just Could Not Blow my Nose

Blowing the nose for most people is a simple, productive task: they blow, mucus exits onto a tissue, and the tissue is disposed. For me, however, blowing was not that productive. Often I would blow with all my might, but little would exit.

I was embarrassed to blow my nose around others, sometimes saving face by enduring the clogged-up nasal feeling for a long time. Other times, I journeyed to a private area where I could blow my nose freely with unmitigated strength until the mucus finally made its exit. When the mucus exited I felt relief of restored breathing through my nose. This respite was usually short-lived, however, as I endured the next battle with this large, thick mucus on a frequent basis, sometimes recurring in hourly intervals.

I did not enjoy blowing my nose forcefully around family members, but it was very uncomfortable and sometimes necessitated such action. At least the mucus came out, which offered temporary relief.

Intuitively, I have always known the importance of being gentle with my nose. Doctors recommend blowing gently to prevent damaging delicate nasal tissue or spreading infection, but I did not know what else to do and could not help myself. My nasal issue was all-consuming and demanded attention. Occasionally when blowing hard the mucus

————— ∞∞∞ —————

d Rather than suggest diminished MCC led to chronic sinusitis, the authors of the article postulated that blockage of the middle meatus led to it. The middle meatus is the opening between the middle and inferior turbinates.

was blood-tinged; other times I accidentally blew air from my nose into my eyes. As a result I would blow softer. These ensuing consequences seemed to slow down my pursuit of mucus extraction, but they did not faze me. My nasal difficulties overpowered any "small complication" in my panged attempts for getting rid of mucus.

Reflecting upon the time immediately following my partial turbinectomy, I should have visited an allergist or ENT specialist or at least enjoyed the fine mist of a saline nasal spray, but I was clueless then, unsure of what to do. After all, I assumed surgery would "solve" my problems and I could not understand why I still experienced so much agony through my nose.

The one reality clear to me was I did not know what to do about my situation.

Little did I realize at the time that I was just beginning the path to self-discovery about my nose, which continues 10 years later at present.

Chapter 2 Reference

1. Berenholz, L., Kessler, A., Sarfati, S., Eviatar, E., & Segal, S. (1998). Chronic sinusitis: A sequela of inferior turbinectomy. *American Journal of Rhinology, 12*, 257-261.

Chapter Three

My Story: The ENS Journey
When My Sinus Problems Persisted

our months after the partial turbinectomy, in December 1997, I returned from Kansas to my hometown of Sauquoit, New York, where I completed the remainder of my undergraduate education. I hoped my nose problems would disappear and I would experience fewer infections, but the opposite was true. Not only did the surgery not improve my rhinosinusitis, but it also exacerbated it. The sinus infections intensified and were just as, if not more, frequent than before. Most of the time I felt more sick than healthy. Nearly all of these infections included an irritated throat, inflammation of my nose and sinuses, and blood-tinged mucus. Depending on the intensity of the symptoms I used over-the-counter medication such as Sudafed® or Benadryl®, while other times I visited my family practice doctor for advice on how to proceed. These visits almost always included a throat culture and sometimes resulted in oral antibiotics.

Regardless of treatment, the duration of my sinus infections seemed to last 2-3 weeks, going through a cycle of symptoms, until the infection finally exited my system—only to return a week or two later. The obvious was apparent to me: no treatment regime seemed to help.

An Allergy Solution

By October 2001, I was determined to discover the root cause of my sinus infections and receive appropriate treatment. I questioned if an allergist could help and requested a referral from my family doctor to visit one.

When I went to a local allergist I underwent extensive testing that demonstrated I had allergies. Keeping this additional reality in mind, I sometimes wonder if treating my allergies could have helped reduce the size of my turbinates rather than my intensive surgery. After all, doctors generally recommend exhausting all minor interventions, such as nasal steroid sprays, antihistamines, allergy shots, or antibiotics prior to recommending surgery.

Between 2001-2004, I received allergy shots for about two and a half years on a weekly, bi-weekly and even tri-weekly basis. Between weeks I waited with anxious anticipation for this shot because I knew it would help me breathe better by thinning some of the unpleasant mucus that seemed otherwise too thick. Allergy shots were beneficial for me, but they were not the panacea.

In 2001, my allergist suggested I take allergy medicine that included a decongestant, Allegra-D®, along with a corticosteroid nasal spray to reduce inflammation of my nasal and sinus membranes. Ultimately the allergy shots seemed to work, but chronic use of a decongestant dried up my nose up for good (or at least I accredited the decongestant for causing such a problem). As I reflect upon that time, however, I realize the decongestant only exacerbated the serious nasal condition I would later learn more about.

Seeking Answers to the Stuffy Sensation

During fall 2002, 5 years after my partial turbinectomy, I began the path to self-discovery about my nose that still continues to this day. While sitting in a classroom of a school psychology graduate course in Oswego, New York, I found myself wanting to blow my nose hard.

I knew the importance of being gentle with my nose, but when it feels like a bowling ball needs to come out or experience partial suffocation through my nasal passages, I blow hard. The only problem is blowing hard did not solve my nasal problems. In fact, it could have made them worse.

Trying to pay attention for the full 3 hours in this graduate course became literally unbearable because my nose demanded constant attention. The dryness felt unbearable and I questioned if my nose then produced any mucus at all. I often became dizzy and lethargic. I knew I had significant issues, but could not pinpoint the problem.

I knew my nasal passages felt chronically stuffy and I understood the symptoms: a sensation of not being able to breathe adequately through my nose, difficulty concentrating, excessive nasal dryness, and occasional blood-tinged mucus.

I visited an ENT doctor at a hospital about one hour from where I reside. The primary symptom I described at that time was my nose felt "stuffy." The doctor looked in my nose and offered a rather grim outlook remarking, "Your nasal passages are wide open, but your turbinates are small—too small." He recommended I try Mucinex®, a tablet containing guaifenesin (which thins mucus, thereby enabling it to better drain). After some doses of Mucinex® I noticed I was able to blow my nose better; to my surprise, there was mucus inside there and I was thankful to be able to blow it out on occasion.

During a series of follow-up visits, the ENT specialist recommended I receive a current CT scan with a coronal (front) view of my nose and sinuses. I had this done in January 2003, roughly six and a half years after my surgery.

Report of my 2003 CT Scan

Post operative changes are noted with fenestration of the maxillary sinuses and partial ethmoidectomy bilaterally. A small amount of residual periosteal thickening is observed with density observed particularly at the base of the maxillary sinuses, slightly greater on the right than the left. The ostiomeatal complexes are patent. *The turbinates have been excised.* The nasal septum is midline. Impression: Post operative changes are noted, mild residual chronic sinusitis is demonstrated.

In short, the above CT scan report stated my turbinates were absent, not just "partially reduced," and I had mild chronic sinusitis. Furthermore, my ethmoid sinuses (sinus cavities between the eyes) were partially removed, even though they were not to have been touched!

The Unhelpful Answer: Further Surgery

Based upon that CT scan, a doctor suggested I might benefit from a surgical procedure known as a bilateral maxillary antrostomy. This procedure consisted of creating a hole in the sinuses by removing bone between my maxillary sinuses (large sinus cavities behind the cheekbone) and natural ostia (drainage holes) to improve mucus drainage. The doctor explained that mucus might get trapped because of blockage between my maxillary sinuses and natural ostia, bacteria would multiply, all of which would lead to infection. He did not suggest this option was a cure-all, but noted I might have about a 30% chance of improvement with this procedure. Suggesting only 30% improvement made me believe he was not particularly optimistic about the procedure. Yet embracing even this glimmer of hope, I decided to go through with it.

However, I incurred a low-grade fever on the day of the operation, which resulted in cancellation of the surgery. While I frequently incurred sinus infections, I rarely contracted a fever. As a believer in God and the ineffable power of Godly intervention, I believe God protected me from this surgery. While I concede that surgery might have offered small improvement to my MCC system, now I realize it would not have improved the breathing difficulties associated with ENS.

Regardless, the next scheduled antrostomy was more than one month away, so I decided to obtain further medical opinion. This added another twist to my already dreadful prognosis: the doctor suggested I had a dry nose and it would *never* get better, and he questioned why such a procedure was recommended in the first place. When he shared his professional opinion with me he appeared angry, but I did not know why. He suggested the best course of action would be environmental modifications that included using a humidifier and buying a hygrometer to measure indoor humidity. He suggested humidity should be kept between 40-50%, which is a comfortable level. So I cancelled the aforementioned surgery and decided to pursue my own research on my nose, and I am glad I did.

The Bittersweet Discovery of Empty Nose Syndrome

It was then I perused the Internet and stumbled upon the phrase "empty nose syndrome" and various terms to describe it. There was no other diagnosis that seemed to perfectly and succinctly describe my condition as well as the following descriptions: the sensation of not getting enough air despite a wide open nasal cavity, nasal dryness, and thick, sticky mucus.

In one sense I was ecstatic to finally discover the condition I seemed to have, but no doctor had yet identified. On the other hand I felt discouraged to learn just how bad this condition really was. I learned that ENS was a terrible problem not only for its physical symptoms, but also because these symptoms had led to a high rate of psychological problems such as depression. One study indicated 52% of people with ENS met clinical criteria for depression, according to the Minnesota Multiphasic Personality Inventory.[1] In fact, Dr. Kern, in a workshop to colleagues, indicated two middle-aged clients committed suicide, perhaps as a direct result of ENS.[2] With an upset stomach or broken leg, pain is temporary. Even with a bad asthma attack you can get relief. With ENS, the difficulties are constant because you breathe twenty-four hours a day.

Sometimes it was difficult to gauge how much of my inadequate nasal breathing was a direct result of thick mucus actually obstructing my breathing, and how much was directly related to paradoxical obstruction. At times it felt great psychologically to know thick mucus could be blown out because it was confirmation that what I was experiencing had an actual basis with tangible evidence.

Striving to blow out mucus through an actual stuffy nose when it was not ready to come out, however, occasionally led me to experience heart pains or soreness in my heart when breathing.

Even when I was able to blow my nose with some success I still experienced shortness of breath (which was odd since so much air was entering my nose). This paradoxical obstruction was constant and also caused shallow breathing in sleep. While adequate sleep is important for our health, many ENS sufferers, including myself, rarely feel well-rested after a good night of sleep.

Perhaps part of the reason no doctor had accurately diagnosed my condition is because much confusion exists in the medical literature regarding diagnosing and treating ENS.[3] Most doctors, or so it seemed, would examine my nose and underestimate the significance of my problems. They would note I had an irritated throat or viral infection, nothing more, and they never seemed to articulate the subjective symptoms I experienced, such as paradoxical obstruction. I felt far worse than they knew.

It was not that ENT doctors were inaccurate about the objective signs I showed because I did have an irritated throat and they might have recognized that. It was not that most ENT doctors did not want to help; each offered piecemeal ideas for remedies, some of which have been beneficial. Rather, these doctors were simply unaware of ENS symptoms.

ENS is mostly invisible, as it is not a physical handicap readily apparent by looking at me. Anyone could look at me but no one would know I have ENS. It can only be determined by a physical examination along with subjective reporting of symptoms. Except for close friends and family, most people do not know I have ENS. Some might recognize I seem to have a nasally voice at times because of thick mucus in my throat, or they might notice I catch numerous colds, or that I blow my nose unnaturally. But that is it. Unless I specifically inform them of my nasal issues, ENS has been a secret, hidden phenomenon. It needs to be revealed and demystified.

Once I learned of ENS, I became desperate for a cure. Like many others with ENS it was hard not to become preoccupied when the issue is *breathing*. One reputable local doctor suggested he would graft some skin and bone from part of my body and then implant it into my nose, thereby creating "artificial turbinates." I was scheduled for a surgery with this ENT doctor in late July 2003, shortly after my wedding, but upon contacting the hospital the night before surgery, as I was instructed to do, I discovered I was not on the docket for surgery. I called the doctor's office the morning of the scheduled surgery and the receptionist told me the doctor was waiting for materials to arrive. Yet the materials never arrived and one year later he referred me to another ENT specialist in Massachusetts whom he suggested was more familiar with ENS.

Apparently, I went through blood work and the emotional preparation for that surgery for nothing. Plus, I took some days off from work, which was tough because at that time I only earned $9.00 per hour at my job and I was preparing for the financial responsibility that comes with marriage.

Preparing for my wedding offered a nice diversion from the physical realities of ENS. How could I possibly be depressed when I had such an exciting future ahead? But the painful reality was that ENS was a chronic problem that would demand my attention if not sooner, then definitely later.

Delaying Real Help while Getting Little

In November 2004, I visited an ENT specialist in Massachusetts. That doctor discussed some treatment options with me. He suggested I could induce swelling in my nasal tissue by creating a rebound effect using an oral decongestant spray[e]. He instructed me to administer 2 sprays into one nostril once per day for 14 days straight, and then the same amount into the other nostril for the following 14 days. He reasoned I would narrow the nasal passages by the rebound effect and consequently feel better. I tried this suggestion but it did not seem to improve my nasal condition; it only made me feel as though I could not breathe as well.

The Massachusetts doctor also discussed surgical techniques including Young's procedure, which consists of closing the nostril for 3 months in an attempt to regenerate nasal tissue.[4] Who would want to experience 3 months of not breathing through one nostril? He also cited how porcine small intestine submucosa (SIS®), a biomaterial from a pig, could

———— ❦ ————

e *Inducing swelling via a rebound effect in the nose leads to unnatural hypertrophy and breakdown of the nasal mucosa, all of which results in increased dryness and diminished nasal airflow sensation. Consequently, this technique is not helpful for an empty nose sufferer.*

be implanted into my nose.[5] The doctor noted, however, there was a good chance this material could fall out because it is so thin and it would require many layers for success; further, he reasoned, there was a high risk of infection. Citing these reasons, during a follow-up visit with this doctor in winter 2005, he recommended more confidently against this procedure as a treatment option. In the meantime, I continued to suffer.

In retrospect, I believe he was simply uncomfortable performing this procedure because he believed it might fail. I am aware of only a small handful of practicing ENT doctors in the United States who perform implant procedures in the nose to improve ENS symptoms. The only American doctors I am aware of who currently perform such procedures include Dr. Houser, Dr. Michael Friedman of Chicago, Dr. Dale Rice of Los Angeles, and Dr. David Slavit of New York City.[6] Clearly, such a procedure constitutes "unchartered territory," as Dr. Houser might put it.

During May 2005, I was still searching for an answer to my nasal plight. A past remedy that seemed helpful in improving my nasal breathing had been allergy shots. Having ENS I would desperately cling to, or blindly grope for, any intervention that might improve my symptoms. I wanted help—and needed it too. I had received allergy shots during earlier years, which were somewhat helpful in alleviating my nasal symptoms.

After two and a half years of allergy shots, I had been without allergy shots for one year and decided again to pursue allergy testing. I went to a doctor who administered a series of painful pricks—more painful than the pricks that felt like mosquito bites from the earlier allergist—and oddly enough he wrote extensively over my skin to mark where he performed the testing. He stated I only had an allergy to dust. Interestingly, I later learned from an ENT specialist that that particular doctor had a bias *against* administering allergy shots. This difficulty in seeking and obtaining help with allergies made it even more difficult to cope with ENS, as his bias meant I went without allergy shots for the remainder of 2005 and into spring 2006. Based upon test results in spring 2006, I was once again a good candidate for allergy shots and could once more experience at least some relief.

Temperature Extremes and ENS

During recent years, car trips seemed long; they often involved lengthy travel in a confined space where air is stagnant and re-circulated. In addition, the car would emit heat in the winter or cold air in the summer, and both tend to dry my nose further. Cold air, in particular, led to a feeling of irritation or mild pain in my nose. It just made rides downright uncomfortable, which leads me to my next point.

The catch-22 for ENS sufferers, particularly for those in the Northeastern United States (which consists of cold, dry winters and warm, humid summers) is how to treat ENS during extreme temperature changes. Most peoples' noses can adapt well to changes in weather, but this is not so for the ENS sufferer.

Winter sports are difficult for ENS sufferers due to the barrage of cold air that immediately penetrates the nasal cavities, which cannot heat or humidify air. ENS sufferers also spend much time in poorly ventilated rooms during winter, and that does not help either.

While entering a warm home on a cold winter day can offer some respite, heat, whether it is from oil, water, electricity, or even the pleasant aroma of a woodstove (though woodstoves emit smoke that exacerbates allergies), further dries out the nose.

Conversely, during a hot, humid summer, allergens such as pollen, dust and mold are widespread and cold, air-conditioned air can contribute to feelings of mild nasal irritation.

All climates considered, however, I believe an ENS sufferer might have the easiest time managing his or her symptoms in a warm, moist climate. It has been my experience that I better manage ENS during the summer in Upstate New York, when it is warm and humid, than in the cold, dry winter. Similarly, Dr. Houser suggests on his website that ENS sufferers might adapt well to a warm, moist climate.[6] The explanation for this position is one can manage his or her allergy symptoms during oppressive heat through allergy medication and injections, but will have much greater difficulty dealing with the onslaught of cold, abrasive air because the nose of an ENS sufferer simply cannot warm or humidify air.

It has been my experience that temperatures between 55-80°F are most comfortable, while temperatures below 55°F seem to irritate my nasal membranes and lungs due to a lack of nasal airflow resistance, which my removed turbinates would have provided. On the other hand, temperatures above 80°F do not offer much improvement to my nasal symptoms. In that respect, perhaps a cool (but not cold) moist climate might also be suitable for an ENS sufferer.

I have always been athletic, but it has been challenging to maintain the same level of stamina as I had before the partial turbinectomy, particularly in cold weather. Research indicates exercise is important to maintain good health because it increases blood flow throughout the body and it increases serotonin levels in the brain, resulting in improved mood. As an ENS sufferer, however, running outside for an extended period of time when temperatures dipped below 55°F almost always irritated my throat and lungs. The turbinates, which had been mostly removed, could not provide the important functions of warming and humidifying air, and my throat and lungs felt the direct effects of prolonged exposure to relatively cold, dry air: irritation and inflamed mucous membranes.

Surprisingly I had the endurance to run the Boilermaker, a 9.3 mile road race in Utica, New York, despite the constant shortness of breath (I ran it in 2002 and 2006, but not other years because of obligations unrelated to my nasal health). It was a major accomplishment to achieve that.

Finally, some ENS sufferers assert they appreciate allergies because it generates more mucus in their noses. That would be true for every ENS sufferer, I believe, if their mucus was watery enough, making it relatively easy to extract. For many people with ENS, however, mucus is thick, which makes it challenging to blow it out and important for them to treat their allergies.

Battling Thick Mucus and Recurrent Infections

Because of ENS, there is often mucus that feels stuck in the back of my nose and upper throat, and I have the desire to frequently gulp or swallow throughout the day. The resulting sensation is notably unpleasant.

I recall visiting restaurants with my girlfriend, who is now my wife, Colleen. Any food that seemed particularly heavy or fatty was difficult for me to keep down. It felt like there were clumps in the back of my throat. Too many times I had to search for the bathroom at the end of a meal, hoping the food would remain in my stomach. Unfortunately, sometimes it did not.

Often, after just part of a day at work, I had so much postnasal drip that conversation was difficult to maintain and I just wanted to go home and rest.

In many respects it seemed mucus was my worst enemy. My nasal experience is in stark contrast to someone whose healthy nose naturally removes about 1-2 liters of mucus per day without notice. The greatly diminished or absent MCC of the empty nose makes it easier for an empty nose sufferer (especially one with rhinosinusitis, such as myself) to get a sinus infection and remarkably harder to get rid of it. That is partly why I, and *some* fellow ENS sufferers, have experienced recurrent viral, bacterial, or fungal infections.

Recurrent infections influence everything, ranging from occupational to social functions, and often last weeks at a time. I spent many days working at a residential home for adults with developmental disabilities, and I would sometimes work overnight shifts or longer. On numerous occasions I had an irritated or mild sore throat, but I had to work to earn money. That was the only option and unfortunate irony: I could either take time off from work to heal from this "sickness" and not earn money, or I could work, risk giving the residents a cold or infection, and earn enough money to support myself and, later, my family. I often opted for the latter, and I was painfully aware when residents contracted a cold or viral infection.

This dilemma continued when I began working in the public school system. I came down with numerous infections during my early public school experiences. There were numerous occasions when I went to school with what felt like a mild sore throat and viral infection that included inflammation of my nasal and sinus membranes. I simply could not get rid of the infecting mucus. A doctor once suggested to me that people miss far more work due to upper respiratory infections such as a sinus infection, than lower respiratory illnesses such as asthma. That was definitely consistent with my experience.

During my practicum in school psychology, which was one day a week, I remember testing students for learning disabilities when I had a cold or viral infection. I recall learning that some of these students were absent shortly after I worked with them, and I felt guilty.

It was not much better during my internship to become a school psychologist. I am certain I missed more days of my internship due to sinus infections than most interns. I recall entering a classroom for emotionally troubled children and one of the children asked why I always sounded stuffy. The teacher jokingly suggested I could respond to this child, "Because I am allergic to you," which I never did, although sometimes I may have felt like saying that!

I tried my best to be considerate of others as I would sometimes use days where I did not feel well to write psychological reports. I like people, but I had to remain a hermit on those days or I would directly expose them. Sometimes I did not have this option, especially if a deadline for testing or major project was imminent.

At one point I pondered whether I might need to leave the profession of school psychology because of ENS. In a *Los Angeles Times* article an ENS sufferer left her paralegal job to work at home and be surrounded by humidifiers, while a chemistry professor had difficulty smelling dangerous fumes because of ENS.[7] Fortunately, with proper medical management, I am confident ENS sufferers can cope and that it will not force people to abandon their professions. I believe there is hope in this area, and I will work at my job as long as I can!

Stress definitely seemed to takes its toll on my physical health by exacerbating the chronic inflammation of my nasal and sinus membranes, and making it hard to get through the day without much buildup of mucus in my throat. At the end of a long day, more than likely, my voice went from sounding clear to more nasally, regardless of how much (or little) I talked.

Even at this writing I have inflammation of my nasal and sinus membranes. This puffy and swollen feeling often makes it more difficult to hold and maintain conversations. Sometimes I just wanted to speak quickly and leave because talking becomes that difficult. During these conversations my voice quickly became nasally sounding.

During one Thanksgiving I just wanted to disappear from sight until I felt better. The fluid and uneven air pressure within my ears were significant. I would have liked a needle to enter my ears and deflate them, which would have made it so much easier to converse. Perhaps I inadvertently blew some fluid in my ears when blowing my nose after saline irrigation. Regardless, Thanksgiving was tough that year and, on various occasions, conversation unbearable. Improved health never looked so good.

An irritated throat has been an accompanying aspect of my recurrent sinus infections. An antibiotic that was sometimes prescribed to fight a bacterial infection would not necessarily rid my system of the throat irritation because it was dryness that led to this irritation.

Frequent past infections, irritated throats, and nasal and sinus inflammation led me to consult ENT doctors many times. I have never been that patient, particularly when it comes to my health, and I guarantee some doctors might have considered me a hypochrondriac—someone who believes he is sick, but is not. Most doctors would generally evaluate me, perform a throat culture test for strep, and then either tell me my throat looks a bit irritated and possibly prescribe an antibiotic, or even suggest I look fine. Yet none of these suggestions helped. I am not a hypochondriac, my issue is real, and it seems few doctors comprehend the subjective realities of ENS. But I will not give up.

People with ENS want help. When presented with an opportunity for help, even through surgery, it is very tempting. However, if these surgeries consist of more turbinate tissue removal, I believe they might make ENS sufferers feel worse, not better. Instead, what we need is real help that will make a substantial improvement for our crippled noses.

Psychological Effects of Coping with ENS

The extent to which ENS affects people on an emotional level varies greatly, with some people reporting it as simply "annoying," while others are more seriously affected.[8] Based upon my conversations with other ENS sufferers, some are upset that doctors might consider them "crazy" or mentally ill, dismissing the role their physical symptoms play in contributing to this state of mind. They believe the constant breathing difficulties and extensive management of it are primary factors leading to depression.

In that respect there is a physiological basis for psychological symptoms that ENS sufferers experience. Most ancient cultures have recognized the connection between satisfying nasal breathing and emotional well-being. Deep nasal breathing results in release of endorphins or "pain killers," while also stimulating the parasympathetic nervous system or "relaxation nervous system." However, when the brain does not receive feedback that nasal breathing is occurring, it alerts the body something is wrong that, in turn, releases stress hormones. Consequently, because of shallow breathing, people with ENS often experience higher levels of stress on a constant basis. This chronic, elevated level of stress is likely to have an adverse effect on a person's life expectancy and emotional well-being, making ENS sufferers more prone to mental health problems. Making matters worse, these emotional symptoms, in turn, are likely to further weaken the immune system.

Given the aforementioned mental health difficulties associated with ENS, a referral for counseling might be appropriate. Counseling would not necessarily remediate the physical pathology, but it could be therapeutic because it allows one to vent about his or her troubles with ENS. Counseling and medical intervention might be recommended together. Cognitive-behavioral therapy is one effective type of counseling. This therapy assumes that thoughts precede behaviors. It focuses on changing the patient's cognitions (thoughts) which might be irrational or hopeless, with the belief that replacing these thoughts with more rational ones will lead to better coping during times of stress.

There have been times where I have questioned, *Am I ever going to get better?* The physical symptoms are constant. However, I do have a strong support system, including my immediate family and faith in Christ, and I believe both serve as buffers against depression.

Other protective and risk factors might also mediate between ENS and depression. An ENS sufferer who has much social support, deep religious faith, an optimistic attitude, and believes he or she can control his or her destiny, to name some factors, might be less likely to develop depression than someone who just lost a loved one, experienced divorce, or feels helpless to control his or her future.

While there are times I have felt confident and strong, I will concede there are times when I cried. I cried because of the severity of this problem and the constant management of it. I cried because I want to have more energy for my wife and children, for people other than myself, but I find myself preoccupied with my nose and depleted of such energy. It seemed selfish to be so consumed with my nose, but I could not avoid it. I wish I could say that I never complained, but I cannot. It is ENS with which I have been dealing and ENS is a difficult condition to endure.

The breathing difficulties of ENS sometimes led to anxiety. It is difficult to think about what one is going to say next when one is battling with how he or she is going to *breathe properly* next, which can be anxiety-provoking. These difficulties in breathing, combined with frequent sinus infections, can lead one to want to avoid social situations. As mentioned, there were times when I preferred to be alone. I enjoy my time with people, but my constant health battles often left me listless and depleted of energy. Sometimes I just needed my space and time to manage ENS.

Why I Will <u>Not</u> Give Up

I would be remiss not to mention my health has improved overall between July 2003 and the present. I understand my nose better now than ever and have learned, over time, many of the medical management strategies used to treat ENS. I have also received valuable implant surgeries that have remedied some of the symptoms.

So I will not give up. I will live life to the fullest. I will overcome ENS the best I can. I ran the Boilermaker twice despite the breathing difficulties. I work a professional job as a school psychologist. I do not let ENS interfere with my family life as I enjoy my beautiful wife and 2 young daughters.

To be sure, I still go through my struggles. Despite interventions in place, breathing out of a dry, seemingly obstructed nose, with irritated nasal and sinus membranes is unpleasant. At times, it seems like my path to discovery on ENS is a never-ending journey with a solution just out of reach. I attempt numerous techniques, some with great success, but other techniques fail as the infections do not go away.

A Fortuitous, but Never-Ending Turn of Events

During the past 3 years I have had my share of differing opinions with ENT doctors regarding how to proceed with my nose. I was frustrated with having various sinus infections throughout the winter and into April 2006. Even the school principal where I work once remarked how "it seemed I had a cold all winter," sometimes playfully joking how I might have given her one on occasion.

In early April 2006 I contacted a local ENT doctor's office with a question: "Because of frequent infections throughout the winter, would it make sense for me to try a low dose oral antibiotic for a month or longer?" Although now I believe the answer was a *no*, there was no answer from that doctor after one and a half weeks. When I called again to follow up on this question and explained my situation politely, the receptionist remarked—in a state of unnecessary defiance—"Dr. X always answers his questions. The office is just very busy." I explained my throat was beet red and I did not know what to do. He never answered.

That doctor's lack of response to the above question, however, could have been a blessing in disguise because the following week I decided to pursue help elsewhere. And I have been seeing another local ENT specialist ever since.

This ENT doctor took his time with me and offered some practical suggestions to improve my health. I greatly appreciated the amount of time he spent with me because I felt like I was being listened to and cared for.

During my first office visit with him he administered a pressure test on my ears and told me I had uneven pressure in my ears, known as disequilibrium. He offered advice on how to blow air into my ears, which would allow my ear pressure to return to a state of equilibrium. To achieve this state I held my breath, plugged my nostrils, and blew air upwards. This doctor remarked it could be helpful to repeat this technique once per hour. He also informed me that my use of a decongestant might be interfering with my sleep as it could be contributing to some anxiety, which seemed correct because decongestants accelerate my heart rate. He recommended using Mucinex® to thin mucus, and Flonase® to reduce inflammation.

Taking Mucinex® and Flonase® consistently made a big difference for the following 5 days. I slept well and felt somewhat well-rested when I awoke in the morning, and I seemed to breathe better and more deeply than in recent memory. It was exciting to notice some improvements as a result of his recommended medical interventions. I was appreciative to enjoy even the *smallest* of improvements.

Unfortunately, I contracted another infection not long thereafter. I could breathe well out of my left nostril, but my right seemed plugged up[f]. It almost seemed as though mucus was trapped in my right nostril. Sometimes, when I could blow mucus out of my right nostril after a long bout of what felt like actual congestion, I felt partial relief. In that respect I was glad to know there was a physical cause to this sensation.

During an office visit with that ENT doctor he examined my nose using a small, black tube called an endoscope. I informed him breathing out my right nostril was worse than breathing out of my left. The right nostril felt obstructed, although the passage was wide open.

As he looked into my nose he remarked that he saw a polyp along my septum and scar tissue blocking my breathing in my right nostril. Since he does not perform surgery anymore, he referred me to another local ENT doctor who he thought would remove this scar tissue. He also said, because scar tissue sometimes grows back, I might need this surgery repeated throughout my life. Clinging to any rationale that could explain why my right nostril felt worse than my left, I believed him. I immediately contacted the other ENT doctor and set up an appointment for June 9, 2006.

---

f I later learned this stuffiness sensation was a direct result of removal of my right inferior turbinate, which led to airflow turbulence in my right nostril, nasal dryness and consequently thick mucus.

At my appointment this ENT doctor looked inside my nose with a flashlight and suggested my primary issue was an "empty nose." He indicated he saw minimal scar tissue. I was crushed. I had hoped for an answer to my complex nasal problem and thought such a surgery could offer at least some relief. I was more confused than ever. Now, I had conflicting medical opinions regarding my nose and I did not know what to do. Upon returning to the other local doctor who recommended scar tissue removal, he suggested how the other doctor did not want to cut obstructing scar tissue because the scar tissue might grow back, or so he explained.

I was confused over these dueling professional opinions and I tried to explain in my own mind the best course of action to take. It was apparent to me that no medical professional up to this point offered a definitive path to take, but merely a piece of the puzzle. Frankly, I felt more confident in the opinion of the doctor who looked at my nose through an endoscope (because of the time, technicality, and overall thoroughness of this examination) than the doctor who looked briefly at my nose via flashlight. I did not know what to do. Because of these conflicting opinions, I wanted a third opinion. I was tired of dealing with conflicting professional opinions in my never-ending journey for nasal relief.

Seeking Help Through Dr. Houser

At this point I was ready to travel any distance for medical opinion and sought help from an ENT doctor familiar with empty nose syndrome: Dr. Steven Houser of Cleveland, Ohio. I was aware Dr. Houser was an authority on ENS because he operates a website that explains an Alloderm® implant tutorial as a surgical treatment for ENS, *www.geocities.com/shouser144/index.html*, and he offers free advice to ENS sufferers on another website at *www.emptynosesyndrome.org*.

Below is an email I sent to him on June 12, 2006:

Dear Dr. Houser:

I am a 27-year-old male with what has been described as "severe atrophic rhinitis" resulting from a septoplasty and partial turbinectomy in 1997. I have been aggressively trying to help my situation by using pulsatile irrigation, Mucinex®, Allegra®, Flonase®, allergy shots, and many of the techniques recommended to help this condition by Dr. Grossan in The Sinus Cure. *My question is this: I recently went to a physician who recommended I have surgery to remove scar tissue that is reportedly partly blocking my breathing through my right nostril. He then suggested I have another surgeon do this procedure, who then suggested I should not undergo any more surgeries on my nose because of my atrophic rhinitis. In other words, I have received two completely different opinions. I have known for years, since the 1997 surgery, that my left nostril breathes much better than my right, but I am unsure why and I don't know what to do. Is removing scar tissue a good or bad idea for someone who has atrophic rhinitis?*

I live in Central New York, but given my level of concern, I would be interested in visiting you at your office for further medical opinion on this topic during this summer or at a later time. I appreciate your help for people with my condition.

Chris Martin

Dr. Houser replied in prompt manner, suggesting I should be very cautious about further surgery that involved tissue removal because of significant tissue loss in the past. He recommended the surgery might be necessary because I reported to him obstructive symptoms, but that he did not know my anatomy and I should be cautious nonetheless. He remarked he would be happy to examine me and to give his office a call, which I did immediately. I was ecstatic at this point just to know he would be willing to examine me. The fact that a doctor who was familiar with, and interested in, treating ENS wanted to see me was very encouraging.

After a series of follow-up phone calls with Dr. Houser's office I learned that I should send him a CT scan, preferably in CD-ROM format, prior to setting up an appointment. I requested my local doctor to write up a script for a CT scan and, after that, I had a CT scan of my nose and sinuses taken on June 21, 2006. As soon as I received a copy of it I mailed it to Dr. Houser. I then waited in anxious anticipation, and Dr. Houser replied on June 29.

Dr. Houser's 2006 Report of my CT Scan

You are missing your inferior and middle turbinates. You have accessory (likely iatrogenic) maxillary antrostomies that do not incorporate the natural ostia. Your ethmoids, frontals, and sphenoids appear clear with minimal thickening at the floor of the maxillary sinuses. Your septum is fairly midline; you do appear to have a very high anterior (front) septal perforation. I would not have any further "scar revision" unless they describe connecting the natural maxillary ostia with the accessory ostia (and then only maybe).

I was thankful for his analysis. In some respects it confirmed what I suspected as a possible cause of my problem: my turbinates were missing. I sent Dr. Houser another email on July 5 and asked, "Since my inferior and middle turbinates are missing based upon my CT scan, could

I schedule an appointment with you for a possible Alloderm®g implant surgery?" Dr. Houser replied that he would be glad to examine me, citing how Alloderm® implants are helpful for "breathing issues," which I seemed to have. He suggested I might need a broad implant along the right septum. He wondered if I was interested in having an office visit first and then, if necessary, an implant at a later time; or if I would try to combine the office visit with an implant the following day to minimize costs and travel, since I was traveling from more than 300 miles away. I opted for the latter.

After receiving this email my wife could sense my excitement. I wore a smile that stretched from one end of my face to the other. *Dr. Houser wanted to see me.* I felt great joy in knowing I would be evaluated and possibly operated on by Dr. Houser.

I contacted Dr. Houser's secretary and provided her with necessary health insurance information. She stated I would not be able to undergo surgery until late August, which I admit then seemed like an eternity, but I was nonetheless very grateful to have this option.

I was unsure if my medical insurance, Excellus Blue Cross Blue Shield, would cover the costs of such a procedure because it was not listed as covered in Blue Cross' policy manual. Since this procedure was uncommon, I feared it might be considered "experimental" and thus not be covered. According to Dr. Houser, the cost of an Alloderm® implant generally ranges from $5,000-$15,000, and he does not have any control over costs, just current procedural terminology (CPT) codes.[9] Dr. Houser's office informed me that Dr. Houser would need to send Blue Cross a letter of medical necessity, and Blue Cross would thereby determine if an Alloderm® implant procedure would be approved.

---

g *Alloderm® is human dermal cells stripped of all tissue taken from a cadaver.*

Dr. Houser had his secretary notify me that, depending upon Blue Cross' response, I might need to visit him first, re-submit for insurance coverage, and then undergo surgery at a later time.

I was anxious to hear from Blue Cross. Getting this close to such a major life goal of improved health was exciting on one hand, but frustrating on the other since a few days of waiting for an answer felt like an eternity. The closer one is to reaching a goal, the more frustrated one is with any impediments. Fortunately, this time nothing blocked my journey to improve my health.

I contacted Blue Cross on a few occasions and, on the morning of August 3, I learned the Alloderm® implant procedure was *approved*. I immediately contacted Dr. Houser's secretary to let her know. I suppose you could say this morning was magical for me as I felt so happy to know this procedure was covered. A light at the end of the tunnel was realized. I was visiting my sister, Robin, and her family in South Carolina, and my happiness showed. It seemed as though every step of this process for an Alloderm® implant surgery fell into place perfectly. I could not have been more pleased. Now the surgery seemed more imminent.

Given all the emotional stress associated with preparing for this surgery, at one point I cried. When stress builds up over time, with my health as a source of anguish for the past 10 years, crying is natural. Learning of this approval meant I could proceed with this surgery, possibly enjoying significant improvement to my nasal health.

Dr. Houser's office then mailed me a variety of booklets regarding nearby hotels, the location of the hospital, as well as appointment and surgery information. My father was generous to drive with me to Cleveland and accompany me during this time. I generally came down with few infections over the summer, but dreadfully I came down with what felt like inflamed nasal and sinus passages during the few days prior to my appointment and surgery. I feared the surgery might be cancelled.

The Office Visit

The office visit with Dr. Houser was on August 21, 2006, at 3:00 PM. As I entered the room to meet Dr. Houser, the nurse asked the reason for my appointment. I explained to him I had come because I have ENS, and he remarked, "You came to the right place. Dr. Houser has operated upon people with ENS from other countries, including someone who came from London." He confirmed what I already knew: I was in good hands.

Dr. Houser met with me and took his time during the office visit, which lasted about an hour and a half. He was courteous and friendly, greeting me with a handshake and answering questions at my pace.

Dr. Houser then examined my turbinates. He investigated my nose gently, concerned about any pain I might have felt. He remarked I had about 10% of my right inferior turbinate remaining, and noted airflow into my right nostril was turbulent, which explained why my right nostril has felt more obstructed than my left. Dr. Houser noted 10% is too small to permit a graft into the right inferior turbinate because the nasolacrimal duct[h] would get in the way; he suggested he usually needs 40-50% to allow a graft to be slid in. Consequently, he suggested I might be a good candidate for a right septal implant.

Dr. Houser performed the cotton test during the office visit. He placed a lengthy, saline-moistened piece of cotton in the region of my nose where the implant might be inserted, which was along the septum in my right nostril since I had so much right inferior turbinate missing. After he placed this cotton into my nose it improved my breathing on

───⊗∞⊗───

h *The nasolacrimal duct is the drainage system from the eyes to the nose.*

the right side, but nasal breathing through my left nostril immediately felt worse. I am not sure how to explain this phenomenon except that the experience of nasal breathing is relative; that is, breathing through my right nostril might seem better only in relation to my left nostril. After Dr. Houser placed this cotton in my nose for about 30 minutes I noticed mucus slowing moving down the back of my throat, and feeling some relief in my nasal breathing. My breathing did not feel improved to perfection, but it did lessen the adverse breathing symptoms associated with ENS. Because the cotton test indicated benefit with my breathing, I was a good candidate for an implant surgery. Dr. Houser explained the surgery would take place under general anesthesia since he would be working deep within my septum. He also explained that I could not have an implant on both sides of my septum during the same operation because that would create a hole in the septum[i].

Dr. Houser asked if I would like a small implant to augment the left inferior turbinate since I had 40% of that turbinate remaining, and I said yes. He placed cotton in my left nasal passage that seemed to improve my breathing.

During the examination, Dr. Houser also observed:

1. I had a hole in my maxillary sinus[j]. He believed this hole was inconsequential because it was small and out of the airway.

2. I had a hole high in the anterior portion of my septum. Dr. Houser believed this was also inconsequential because it was small and out of the airway.

---

i *The septum consists of thin bone and cartilage, which is why an implant on both sides during the same operation might lead to a hole in it. However, it might be possible to implant each side of the septum during different surgeries without creating a hole.*

j *The doctor created a hole in my maxillary sinus in order to enable better draining of mucus.*

3. I had rhinosinusitis, not just sinusitis, due to inflammation of my nose and sinuses.

Dr. Houser's Grading of my Turbinates

Middle turbinates absent (stubs remain); 40% of left inferior turbinate remains; 10% of right inferior turbinate remains.

Let me reflect for a moment on my nasal anatomy based upon Dr. Houser's exam, his analysis of my CT scan, and the 2003 CT scan. The 1997 partial turbinectomy and septoplasty left me in the following state:

I had only 10% of my middle turbinates and right inferior turbinate remaining; I had 40% of my left inferior turbinate remaining; I had a hole high on my septum; I had a hole in my maxillary sinus; and my ethmoid sinuses were partly removed.

Clearly, far more was removed than stated by the procedures, *partial turbinectomy* and *septoplasty*.

Toward the end of the office visit Dr. Houser showed me two biomaterials, Alloderm® and SIS®, that have been suggested as possible implant materials for ENS. The Alloderm® was considerably thicker than SIS®. He remarked how he prefers Alloderm® because SIS® might "crinkle like a newspaper" if damaged, whereas Alloderm® is more durable.

The Good Surgery

The following day, Tuesday, August 22, 2006, was my surgery. Before surgery a nurse stated offhandedly that Dr. Houser gets excellent results post-surgery. This was just another confirmation of what I already knew. I was nervous before this surgery, but comforted in knowing Dr. Houser was the one to operate on me. As I was wheeled into the operating room at about 10:45 AM, I noticed Dr. Houser off to the side looking at a large screen, probably preparing for the surgery. The assistants helped me onto a platform, and before I knew it I was fast asleep.

I was awakened around 3:00 PM by a nurse who informed me Dr. Houser would be checking on me soon. As I am sure most people who have undergone surgery would agree, general anesthesia left me feeling quite groggy, so the rest of this day was somewhat of a blur. I had to be physically assisted walking to the car after surgery, and I rested for the remainder of the day. I did have nasal packing in my right nostril, but not my left. I did not sleep well that night because of it.

The following day, Wednesday, August 23, I had a follow-up visit with Dr. Houser. He examined my nose and carefully removed the packing; in contrast to the past experience with the ENT doctor who performed my partial turbinectomy, here again was a pleasant, or at least not too aversive, experience. Dr. Houser answered many of my questions and instructed me not to blow my nose for at least 2 weeks, not to engage in rigorous exercise for 3 weeks, or do pulsatile irrigation for a month. He did, however, suggest I could use a saline nasal spray as long as I did not jam it into the implant by spraying directly onto that area. He also indicated I would likely recognize the permanent effects to my nasal breathing about 6 weeks after surgery.

On the following page are photos looking directly inside my nose that Dr. Houser took immediately before and after surgery. As you view the photos, imagine I am looking directly at you.

My Nose before Surgery

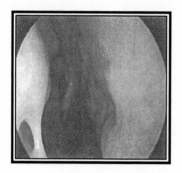 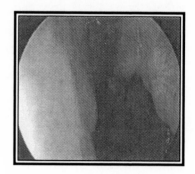

Figure 2. Right Nostril　　*Septum*　　*Figure 3. Left Nostril*

My Nose after Surgery

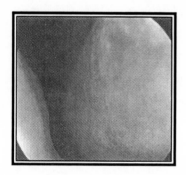 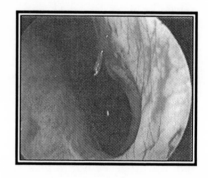

Figure 4. Right Nostril　　*Septum*　　*Figure 5. Left Nostril*

Notice how the right septum and left inferior turbinate are bulkier after surgery, thereby providing greater nasal airflow resistance.

After the Surgery

As my father and I drove home on August 23 from Cleveland to Sauquoit, I was still early in the recovery. Patients in a post-surgical state often have a lot of crusting as their noses heal. I sensed crusts in one nostril of my nose, almost to the point of not being able to breathe through it. Through careful extraction, the crusting finally exited my nose.

I was very anxious regarding my post-operative condition and reported to Dr. Houser via email that I had a white piece hanging toward the back of my nose, concerned I might have moved the implant by wiggling my nose on the drive home. He replied it was likely a stitch and that I would not be able to remove the implant unless I literally removed every single stitch and pulled the implant out, which he light-heartedly implied I should not do.

The following day I sent Dr. Houser another naïve question, although important to me at the time. I informed him I could see a white piece hanging from inside my nose and questioned if this could possibly be Alloderm®. He replied that my implant was submucosal (beneath the mucous layer) and therefore could not be seen.

Upon arriving home I spent part of the first evening enjoying the fresh, outdoor air. As my wife and daughters were in the backyard, I was in the front yard. I noticed a Monarch butterfly on a flower in the grass, which had recently hatched out. At first it started to flutter but was weak. Then, as it practiced its fluttering, it gradually became stronger until it flew away with ease. Seeing this butterfly gradually become stronger seemed like a perfect metaphor for what I was experiencing at the time. This butterfly represented to me freedom from past ills, such as ENS. I believed I would improve and I had hope. The butterfly confirmed it.

The first two weeks following surgery were an interesting time. For some nasal surgeries, congestion is a predictable outcome for the initial weeks after surgery. Interestingly, I must have had more actual congestion during the first few weeks post-surgery than I had in the past 10 years!

Having a runny nose for a few days, for example, was a fascinating experience because I could not have had one if I wanted it in the prior 10 years due to chronic nasal dryness.

Four days after the surgery I was resting one evening and noticed how my nose and lungs worked together in harmony; it was the best feeling in the world! This feeling was particularly noticeable when I laid on my left side, with my right nostril enjoying the upper half. Consequently, sleep became more restful. My sleep was much improved for the following month and a half because I could breathe more deeply. My wife similarly observed I seemed to be less awake in the night because of my nose, and my nasal blowing habits were gentler. I would not awaken in the middle of the night and blow with all my might, for example.

Another benefit of the surgery was airflow seemed less harsh on my lungs because of increased nasal airflow resistance. The air entering my nose, even in cold weather, seemed moister and therefore not as harsh on my lungs.

Another positive result of the surgery was I had more mucus in my nose. Narrowing the nasal passage via an Alloderm® implant appeared to have improved the moisture content in my nose. Dr. Houser reported every person who received this implant has reported improvement in moisture. When I blew my nose, mucus exited with greater ease. An increase in mucus production and moisture led me to believe my nasal and sinus passages would become less irritated and maybe my MCC system would even work better.

I could also smell better because airflow was more orderly and directed toward my olfactory nerves, particularly those in my right nostril. Although I still had a stronger sense of smell in my left nostril than my right, my overall sense of smell was improved.

While the first surgery was not a panacea, it was an improvement and, perhaps just as important, it gave me hope. It has also made me less eager to undergo surgery for this problem, which is contrary to how I felt before the surgery; ENS still requires management, such as saline irrigation, but it has not been as challenging to cope with.

After some months passed I felt some mild regression in symptoms since the surgery, such as increased dryness in my nose and less restful sleep, but overall I was still improved since before the surgery. As the blood vessels incorporated into the Alloderm® (causing the Alloderm® to shrink in size as the air bubbles filled in), the positive effects in breathing also became less noticeable, but again I still experienced an overall improvement in breathing compared to my condition before surgery.

Dr. Houser noted my implant looked exactly as desired during an office visit in December 2006 and stated that further augmentation would bring me further relief. Consequently, I underwent a second Alloderm® implant operation on February 20, 2007.

It is 2 months after the second implant as of this writing and this implant seems to have further helped. I recently had a cold and mucus production was much more than before the implants. The cold only lasted about 8 days, whereas it might have lasted 2-3 weeks before the implants. This increased nasal resistance also allows me to inspire cold, dry air even more comfortably now. Breathing is still not completely natural, but it is an improvement.

It is clear these implants have helped me cope more effectively with ENS and, if you are an ENS sufferer and your insurance covers it, I highly recommend this particular operation and ENT doctor. The implants have lessened stress associated with ENS. Now that I have received help, I want to advocate on behalf of others suffering from ENS. I know how tough ENS can be. I also believe there is hope.

Chapter 3 References

1. Moore, E.J., & Kern, E.B. (2001). Atrophic Rhinitis: A review of 242 cases. *American Journal of Rhinology*, 15, 355-361.

2. Kern, E.B. (2006, audioclip). *Click here to listen to Dr. Kern's ENS Lecture.* Retrieved November 24, 2006, from the Empty Nose Syndrome Association Web site: *www.emptynosesyndrome.org.*

3. Houser, S.M. (2004, September). *Empty Nose Syndrome Associated with Middle Turbinate Resection.* Poster Presented at the meeting of the American Rhinological Society, New York.

4. Young, A. (1971). Closure of the nostril in atrophic rhinitis. *Journal of Laryngology and Otology*, 81, 515-524.

5. Houser, S.M. (2006a). *Frequently Asked Questions.* Retrieved November 24, 2006, from Rhinology/Allergy Pages Web site: *www.geocities.com/shouser144/ens5.html.*

6. Houser, S.M. (2006b). *Empty Nose Syndrome: please read all theses pages if you have an interest in this topic.* Retrieved November 24, 2006, from Rhinology/Allergy Pages Web site: *www.geocities.com/shouser144/empty.html.*

7. Zitner, A. (2001, May 10). Sniffing at Empty Nose Idea. *Los Angeles Times*, p. A.1.

8. Houser, S.M. (2006c). Empty nose syndrome associated with middle turbinate resection. *Otolaryngology - Head and Neck Surgery*, 135, 972-973.

9. Houser, S.M. (2006a). *Frequently Asked Questions.* Retrieved November 24, 2006, from Rhinology/Allergy Pages Web site: *www.geocities.com/shouser144/ens5.html.*

Chapter Four

What Exactly is Empty Nose Syndrome?

Now that you have insight into what an ENS sufferer experiences, it would be helpful to explain the anatomical and physiological basis of ENS. There are clear reasons I have experienced many of the problems discussed, and hopefully all my experiences will come together and make sense as you delve into the next section. First, below is a definition of empty nose syndrome:

Definition of Empty Nose Syndrome

Empty nose syndrome (ENS) is a cluster of symptoms in individuals who had a turbinate reduction or excision surgery that resulted in removal of too much turbinate tissue, leaving the nose "empty" or wide open and the turbinates unable to function properly. This syndrome is considered to be highly variable and poorly defined.[1] A feeling of not getting enough air, despite the nasal cavity being wide open, is a unique and perplexing symptom of ENS called paradoxical obstruction. Other symptoms include chronic nasal dryness, difficulty concentrating, frequent headaches, increased pulmonary reactivity to volatile compounds or airborne irritants, decreased ventilation of the lungs, a diminished sense of smell, thick, sticky mucus, shallow sleep, minor nosebleeds, fatigue, and sometimes crusting, recurrent sinus infections and/or sinus pain or pressure, all of which might lead to anxiety and depression.

The Turbinates: How Form Fits Function

It is important to understand the various roles of the turbinates and how form fits function to better understand ENS.

The turbinates consist of bone (also referred to as nasal concha) sandwiched between mucous layers, and they are rich in blood vessels and nerve endings. The outer portion is thick with significant mucus-producing capabilities. Turbinate tissue removal leads to destruction of much nasal mucosa and scar tissue formation, resulting in fewer cilia. Due to fewer cilia and impaired cilia functioning, mucus builds up and bacteria, viruses, mold, and fungi stay in place rather than being properly disposed of for destruction by stomach acid.

The turbinates consist of inferior[k], middle, superior, and in some instances, supreme[l].

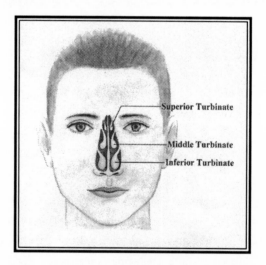

Figure 6. Front View of Turbinates

k *The inferior turbinates are similar in size to the index finger and the middle turbinates are similar in size to the pinky finger. The superior and supreme turbinates are much smaller.*
l *Some people have a supreme turbinate that is tiny and situated above the superior turbinate.*

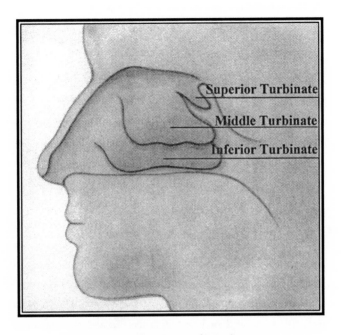

Figure 7. Side View of Turbinates

The turbinates serve many important functions for the 18,000 liters of air we breathe and 1-2 liters of mucus that goes through our nose and sinuses each day, including:

1. *Directing airflow.* The nose directs airflow in an orderly pattern so that air is experienced throughout all regions of the nose. The groove-like air space between the turbinates and between the inferior turbinate and nasal floor are called "meatuses," which help direct airflow in an orderly direction and at the right velocity.

2. *Providing nasal airflow resistance.* The nose provides greater than 50% of resistance in overall airflow to our lungs, ensuring optimal lung functioning. This resistance prepares inspired air at the right temperature and humidity for the lungs to ensure that optimal respiration[m] occurs at the alveoli[n] level of the lungs[o].

3. *Containing nerve cells.* Laminar airflow strikes the nasal mucosa, which is embedded with trigeminal receptors (nerve receptors that detect airflow motion and temperature) and these nerve cells tell the brain you are breathing. There is also a possibility that direct nerve damage or poor re-growth of nerve cells contributes to reduced recognition of airflow.

4. *Humidifying* the air we breathe. The turbinates help moisten the air we inspire so it is near 100% humidity by the time it reaches our lungs. Such moisture also helps thin mucus.

5. *Warming* the air we breathe. Turbinates help warm air not only by providing nasal airflow resistance, but also the larger and lower turbinate (the inferior turbinate, which is rich in blood vessels) has significant expanding (to decrease cold air intake) and contracting (to allow more air to enter our nose) capabilities. Specifically, the anterior portion of the inferior and middle turbinates plays a significant role in directing and warming air upon inspiration, while the posterior (back) end of the inferior turbinates plays an important role in directing air and retaining nasal moisture and warmth upon expiration. These functions ensure air is near body temperature by the time it reaches our lungs.

---

m Breathing is air passing through the upper and lower airways to cells, while respiration is the process of bringing oxygen to every cell in the body and removing carbon dioxide from tissues and organs.

n Alveoli are small hollow cavities in the lungs that ensure proper gas (oxygen-carbon dioxide) exchange with the blood.

o Given breathing difficulties, ENS sufferers are generally mouth breathers. However, nasal breathing results in 10-20% more oxygen uptake than mouth breathing.[2]

6. *Filtering* the air we breathe. The turbinates provide much surface area to allow infectious particles to strike them, entrapping them in mucus, which is swept into the pharynx where it is harmlessly swallowed.

7. *Smelling* the air we breathe. The turbinates project a small amount of air, 10% or less, toward the superior turbinates where olfactory bulbs are present that help detect smell.

8. *Swelling.* The turbinates swell on one side of the nose while the other side constricts every 2-4 hours, a process known as the nasal cycle. Consequently, we usually breathe through only one side of the nose at a time while the other side relaxes. The nasal cycle also helps prevent bedsores. During sleep, the dependent inferior turbinate fills up with blood, pushing gently against the septum, thus causing the person to roll without waking. This process might happen 50 times per night.

So what exactly is the phenomenon of "paradoxical nasal obstruction," a puzzling symptom experienced by ENS sufferers? It is the sensation that one is not breathing adequately, while in actuality they are inspiring large amounts of air. Some might state their noses feel "stuffy," as I did, or "too open."

To understand its physiological origin, it is important to understand the aerodynamics of the nose.

Bernoulli's Principle helps explain airflow speed through the nose. This principle states that as the velocity of fluid increases, its pressure decreases. Applying this principle to the nose suggests the highest velocity rates will be found at the narrowest regions of the nose, with wider regions having lower velocity. One study found that inspiratory velocity is greatest at the nasal valve region (6-18 meters/second), decreases in the main passage (2 meters/second) and then increases again as air reaches the nasopharynx (3 meters/second). [3]

The nasal valve area is near the front of the nose and it is the narrowest portion of the nasal passage, thereby providing a significant amount of nasal airflow resistance, while the nasopharynx is much wider and it is behind the nose where it meets the upper throat. The nasal valve region is also a prime site of nasal airflow sensation. Here, the heads of the inferior turbinates, with their significant expanding and contracting abilities, direct airflow like your thumb on a water hose. Put your thumb on the end of a hose and you will notice water reaches the far end. Take it off and, although the opening is wide open, the water drips at your feet. In the same manner, someone whose anterior portions of his or her inferior turbinates are intact can enjoy a deeper, more satisfying breath than someone without them.

Removal of turbinates leads to turbulent inspired airflow. Grutzenmacher, Lang and Mlynski suggest that normal airflow consists of air entering the nose in an orderly fashion, generally stimulating the nerve cells of most regions of the nose.[4] However, Grutzenmacher et al. and Proetz suggest that when inferior turbinates are removed airflow primarily tends to be directed in haphazard fashion toward lower portions of the nose, with some of the air not properly stimulating much of the nose.[5] When middle (or inferior and middle) turbinates are removed, the air enters in a zigzag direction.

With these explanations in mind, various factors contribute to this sensation of paradoxical obstruction when turbinates are removed[p]:

———∞∞∞———

p *The factors contributing to paradoxical nasal obstruction might interact in a synergistic manner. That is, the interaction of these factors might create a combined effect that is greater than the sum of their individual effects.*

✦ Airflow becomes too turbulent and does not flow through all regions of the nose, resulting in air being conducted less efficiently from the nose to the lungs and a lack of nasal mucosa stimulation.

✦ The lack of stimulation to the nasal mucosa, which are embedded with trigeminal receptors, registers in the brain as a lack of air entering the nose. Nerve damage or poor re-growth of nerve cells might further lead to a lack of airflow recognition.

✦ Due to reduced capacity for humidifying, filtering and heating air, the quality of air is greatly diminished as it reaches the lungs, resulting in inefficient gas-exchange in the alveoli of the lungs.

✦ Diminished nasal airflow resistance weakens the elasticity (flexibility) of the lungs and consequently decreases expansion of the lungs.

✦ Air not properly ventilating all parts of the nose, particularly the upper cavities, results in a diminished sense of smell. The olfactory nervous system is responsible for smell. Because of the interaction between the olfactory and trigeminal nerves, a weakened sense of smell further decreases the sensation of airflow motion through the nose.

✦ Chronic nasal dryness leads to decreased blood supply to the nasal mucosa. Such dryness also leads to decreased nasal cilia functioning, decreased mucus production and, among other problems, decreased nasal sensations and reflexes.

There is a direct reflex between the nose and lungs known as the nasal-bronchiole reflex. An example of this reflex is when nerve cells in the nose detect smooth, orderly air entering it, the lungs relax and allow for deep inhalation.[6-9] Conversely, if the nose does not detect orderly airflow the lungs become more tense and pulmonary breathing is increasingly shallow. With ENS, the natural harmony of breathing between the nose, mouth, and lungs is impaired. Consequently, people with untreated ENS are at greater risk for pulmonary problems, such as bronchitis or asthma.

There is also a direct reflex between the nose and heart known as the nasal-cardiac reflex.[10-11] For example, when the nose detects airflow the heartbeat slows; when the nose does not detect airflow, the heartbeat accelerates. A weakened nasal-cardiac reflex might help explain why people with ENS are at increased risk for high blood pressure.

These reflexes, in combination with proper nasal airflow resistance, ensure optimal functioning of the lungs and heart.[12-13]

Removal of turbinates also leads to a diminished ability for the nose to heat and humidify air as demonstrated in one article. Wolf, Naftali, Schroter, and Elad revealed that removal of the inferior turbinates might reduce the heat and water vapor content in the nose by 16%, removal of the middle turbinates might reduce heat and water vapor content by 12%, and removal of both turbinates might reduce heat and water vapor content by 23%.[14] They suggest these losses could be partially recovered by 6% through reconstructive surgery, such as an Alloderm® implant. In other words, while the ability to heat and moisturize inspired air will be absent with removed turbinates (as a result of removed blood vessels and glands), this study finds these functions can be partially recovered through reconstructive surgery.

Physical Symptoms of ENS

• A feeling of never getting enough air, as if in a chronic state of dyspnea, due to shortness of breath through the nose and weakened ventilation of the lungs, which in turns leads to difficulty concentrating, causing headaches and a

---

Physical Symptoms of ENS (cont.)

tendency to hyperventilate at real or perceived external pressures. Guye of Amsterdam proposed the term "aprosexia nasalis," meaning a lack of memory and inability to concentrate as a consequence of enlarged adenoids (tissue deep within the nose) that were obstructing breathing.[15] This term might also be applied to ENS sufferers.

• A lack of deep breathing or "sleep-disordered" breathing often leads to shallow, unrestful sleep, as many people with ENS will wake up not feeling rested in the morning; some also have frequent nightmares. Sometimes this shallow breathing, combined with dry nasal passages, can lead to snoring or even sleep apnea. A sleep specialist, often concerned with sleep apnea, might find ENS patients difficult to understand because they snore loudly and experience shallow sleep, but they might not show signs of sleep apnea. Consequently, the specialist might refer an ENS patient for anxiety or depression because of his or her poor sleep which is often associated with these mental health issues, although his or her poor sleep is in part a direct result of shallow breathing.

• Chronic nasal dryness.

• Dry pharyngitis.

• Dry laryngitis and accompanying voice difficulties.

• Thick, sticky mucus.

• Occasional crusting.

• Too little or, in some instances, too much mucus production.

• A diminished sense of smell and/or taste.

• Sinus pain or pressure.

• Minor nosebleeds or blood-tinged mucus.

• Unequal ear pressure, fluid in the ears, and/or patulous eustachian tubes.

• Foul-smelling odors from the nose.

• Increased pulmonary reactivity to volatile compounds (such as gasoline or paint) or airborne irritants (such as perfume).

Psychological Symptoms of ENS

◆ Anxiety

◆ Depression

◆ Social avoidance

◆ Panic disorder

Proposed classification system for ENS:
IT, MT and Both

Dr. Houser proposed 3 subtypes of ENS to delineate symptoms associated with each type, thereby guiding their respective treatments.

Dr. Houser's Proposed Subtypes of ENS[15]

1. ENS-IT: part or total inferior turbinate excision.

2. ENS-MT: part or total middle turbinate excision.

3. ENS-Both: both inferior and middle turbinates are at least partially excised.

ENS-IT is considered the most prevalent subtype and therefore ENT physicians somewhat agree upon its existence. This subtype is most noted for paradoxical obstruction, and the patient might be viewed by his or her doctor as somewhat of a hypochondriac because his or her nasal airways look open, even though he or she complains of obstruction in nasal breathing. These patients also develop crusting, thick mucus, a diminished sense of smell (due to inspired airflow along the nasal floor), and they might occasionally experience mild pain. People with ENS-IT claim they breathe better during an upper respiratory infection, such as a cold.

Interestingly, some people who had a complete removal of their inferior turbinates will not report ENS symptoms, while others with only a partial removal will report symptoms. The reason for conflicting reports between ENS patients is unclear; it is possible this difference relates to a difference in nasal airflow. There is also a possibility this difference might relate to a variance in their perception of breathing despite similar breathing difficulties, as some might remain in denial of this breathing anomaly.

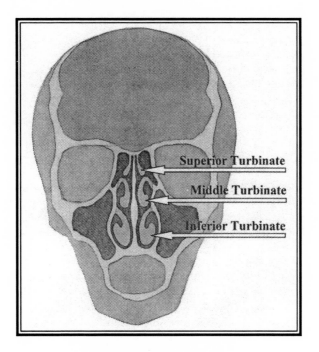

Figure 8. Normal CT Scan

Editor's note: Figures 8-11 of CT scans are not exact anatomic representations, but are for illustrative purposes only.

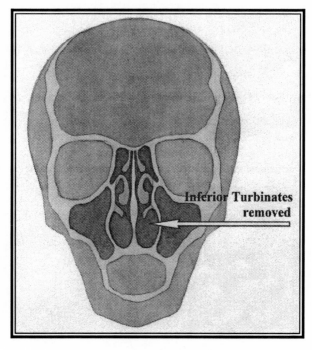

Figure 9. CT Scan with Inferior Turbinates Removed
(ENS-IT)

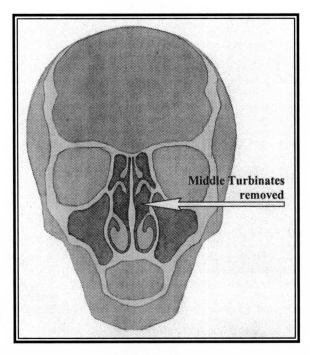

*Figure 10. CT Scan with Middle Turbinates Removed
(ENS-MT)*

ENS-MT is less agreed upon among ENT doctors and middle turbinate reductions are still considered a standard medical procedure today. People with ENS-MT might have sinus pain and pressure, given the middle turbinate's position between the eyes and high up in the sinuses. According to Dr. Houser, these patients might also describe some nasal obstruction, mild nasal crusting, and a decreased sense of smell, although these latter problems are less severe than for those with ENS-IT.

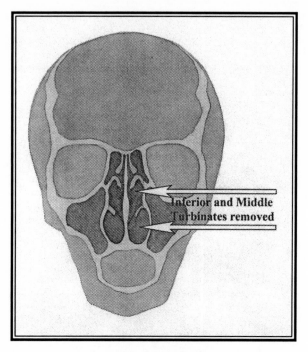

Figure 11. CT Scan with Inferior and Middle Turbinates Removed (ENS-Both)

ENS-Both (the subtype that represents my condition) consists of removal of both inferior and middle turbinates, and includes all the symptoms of the prior two subtypes. Dr. Houser described this subtype as most associated with the concept of a "nasal cripple," someone literally disabled by surgery.[16] People with this type tend to have symptoms associated with ENS-IT and ENS-MT.

Most diagnoses regarding ENS involve the inferior and middle turbinates, but not the superior turbinates. Dr. Houser indicated that normally the superior turbinates remain intact among his ENS patients. Because the superior turbinates are small and outside of the airway, cutting them might not make a big difference in patient symptoms. However, the superior turbinates do contain olfactory tissue and their removal might reduce a patient's sense of smell.

Empty Nose Syndrome or Atrophic Rhinitis?

It is important to clarify the differences between empty nose syndrome (ENS) and atrophic rhinitis since these two terms are often used interchangeably, but represent distinctly different disorders. ENS is different from, and if managed properly, can prevent the development of atrophic rhinitis.

Atrophic rhinitis was first coined by Dr. Bernhard Fraenkel in 1876 to describe fetor (odor from the nose), crusting, and atrophy of inner nasal structures, with reports of it dating back to ancient times.[17, 19] Atrophic rhinitis is an inflammatory, degenerative disease involving total dysfunction of the remaining nasal mucosa, and it is often accompanied by enlarged nasal space, nasal crusting, nosebleeds, and a foul-smelling odor (which patients are not aware of due to their loss or diminished sense of smell, but it is apparent to everyone around them).

Two terms used interchangeably with atrophic rhinitis are rhinitis sicca and ozena.

Rhinitis sicca is a dry nose that has little or no ability to produce mucus, and it usually includes hypertrophy of the nasal mucosa. ENS, in some instances, can be similar or even tantamount to rhinitis sicca.

Ozena, a Greek term meaning stench, is a late stage of atrophic rhinitis that includes progressive atrophy (versus hypertrophy that is seen with rhinitis sicca and the early stages of atrophic rhinitis) of the submucous membrane and turbinate bone. It often follows long-term hypertrophy of the nasal mucosa. Nasal crusting, discharge, and fetor are common symptoms of ozena, and perhaps more common than among patients with an early stage of atrophic rhinitis. Klebsiella ozaenae and Bacillus foetidus are bacteria reported to be present in patients with ozena.

For many years people with ENS, including myself, have been wrongly labeled as having secondary atrophic rhinitis, with *secondary* meaning that the atrophic rhinitis was iatrogenic, or directly caused by medical treatment. By contrast, primary atrophic rhinitis might have been caused by unknown etiology such as infections, nutritional deficiencies, chronic sinusitis, or even genetics, but not surgery. Given the increased use of antibiotics and improved oral hygiene over the past century, the incidence of primary atrophic rhinitis appears to have diminished significantly, particularly in the Western world, though it is still commonly found in developing countries such as India.[17-18]

An aging nose among the elderly might create mild symptoms of ENS (or atrophic rhinitis) due to age-related shriveling of the remaining turbinates and subsequent enlargement of the nasal cavities. That is why when I suggested I had "atrophic rhinitis," a local ENT doctor responded I was too young to have it.

Many years of ENS can result in the remaining nasal mucosa becoming increasingly drier, which might cause it to become metaplastic[q] (changing from one cell type to another, in this case from ciliated epithelium to squamous, nonciliated epithelium) and atrophic, at which point the problem can be correctly diagnosed as atrophic rhinitis. Nevertheless, an ENS sufferer might still show some small patches of metaplasia in the mucous membrane, but these do not encompass the entire nasal mucosa, the latter of which indicates atrophic rhinitis.

---

q *Crusting is usually noted in mucous membranes that have become metaplastic. The main way to determine if metaplasia of the mucosa has occurred is through biopsy. A small piece of mucosa is removed and sent to a lab to assess the cilia.*

While ENS can develop into atrophic rhinitis, it is misleading to suggest ENS begins as atrophic rhinitis or that it always implies atrophy because people with ENS experience symptoms of loss of airflow sensation immediately after turbinate surgeries, regardless of whether they experience atrophy of the nasal mucosa. The latter might take several years to develop.

Furthermore, Dr. Cottle contended some people with nasal mucosal atrophy might never develop crusts, fetor, or anosmia[r]. Yet he observed that patients without full blown atrophic rhinitis might have, and doctors should be actively looking for, the following signs:[20]

- Thin, dry pale patches of mucous membrane where metaplastic changes had occurred.
- Sticky mucosal secretions.
- Small bleeding.
- Increase in nasal space.

During his career Dr. Houser has evaluated a large number of ENS patients and, as of December 2006, has only evaluated 2 cases of atrophic rhinitis.

A doctor once wrote to another ENT doctor suggesting I had "severe atrophic rhinitis, resulting in ENS." As one might glean from the prior discussion, this statement is incorrect. A more accurate statement would have been I had "ENS that could potentially develop into atrophic rhinitis if left untreated."

---

r *Anosmia is the loss of sense of smell while a related term, hyposmia, is a decrease in the ability to smell.*

Chapter 4 References

1. Houser, S.M. (2006c). Empty nose syndrome associated with middle turbinate resection. *Otolaryngology—Head and Neck Surgery*, 135, 972-973.

2. Cottle, M.H. (1972). Nasal breathing pressures and cardio-pulmonary illness. *Eye, Ear, Nose and Throat Monthly*, 51, 331-340.

3. Girardin, M., Bilgen, E., & Arbour, P. (1983). Experimental study of velocity in a human nasal fossa by laser anemometry. *Annals of Otology, Rhinology, and Laryngology*, 92, 231-236.

4. Grutzenmacher, S., Lang, C., & Mlynski, G. (2003). The combination of acoustic rhinometry, rhinoresistometry and flow simulation in noses before and after turbinate surgery: A model study. *Journal for Otorhinolaryngology and its Related Specialties*, 65, 341-347.

5. Proetz, A.W. (1951). Air currents in the upper-respiratory tract and their clinical importance. *Annals of Otology, Rhinology, & Laryngology*, 60, 439-467.

6. Fontanari, P., Burnet, H., Zattara-Hartmann, M.C., & Jammes, Y. (1996). Changes in airways resistance induced by nasal inhalation of cold dry, dry, or moist air in normal individuals. *Journal of Applied Physiology*, 81, 1739-1743.

7. Widdicombe, J.G. (1996). Neuroregulation of the nose and bronchi. *Clinical Experimental Allergy*, 26, 32-35.

8. Kratschmer, F. (2001). On reflexes from the nasal mucous membrane on respiration and circulation. *Respiratory Physiology*, 127, 93-104.

9. Hens, G., & Hellings, P.W. (2006). The nose: the gatekeeper and trigger of bronchial disease. *Rhinology*, 44, 179-187.

10. Betlejewski, S., Betlejewski, A., Burduk, D., & Owczarek, A. (2003). Nasal-cardiac reflex. *Otolaryngologia Polska*, 57, 613-618.

11. Baxandall, M.L. (1988). The nasocardiac reflex. *Anaesthesia*, 43, 480-481.

12. Butler, J. (1960). The work of breathing through the nose. *Clinical Science*, 19, 55-62.

13. Edison, B.D. & Kerth, J.D. (1973). Tonsilloadenoid hypertrophy resulting in cor pulmonale. *Archives of Otolaryngology*, 98, 205-207.

14. Wolf, M., Naftali, S., Schroter, R.C., & Elad, D. (2004). Air-conditioning characteristics of the human nose. *The Journal of Laryngology and Otology*, 118, 87-92.

15. *Adenoid* Problem. Retrieved November 24, 2006, from the Old and Sold Antiques Digest Web site: *www.oldandsold.com/articles35/common-cold-14.shtml.*

16. Houser, S.M. (2006c). Empty nose syndrome associated with middle turbinate resection. *Otolaryngology - Head and Neck Surgery,* 135, 972-973.

17. Moore, E.J., & Kern, E.B. (2001). Atrophic Rhinitis: A review of 242 cases. *American Journal of Rhinology,* 15, 355-361.

18. Garcia, G.J.M., Martins, D.A., Bailie, N., & Kimbell, J.S. (2004). Investigations of atrophic rhinitis in humans using computational fluid dynamics models of the nasal passages. *CIIT Centers for Health Research.*

19. Cowan, A., Ryan, M.W., & Quinn, Jr., F.B. (2005, March). *Atrophic Rhinitis.* Paper Presented at the meeting of the Grand Rounds Presentation, UTMB, Department of Otolaryngology, Galveston.

20. Cottle, M.H. (1958). Nasal atrophy, atrophic rhinitis, ozena: medical and surgical treatment. *Journal of the International College of Surgeons,* 29, 472-484.

Chapter Five

Commentary on Turbinate Surgeries

Turbinate reduction and removal procedures have been performed for more than 100 years, but not without controversy. These procedures are often done in conjunction with other nasal or sinus surgeries (such as a septoplasty or ethmoidectomy) and generally consist of removing an enlarged turbinate bone and/or mucosa.

Numerous turbinate reduction procedures exist at present, all with respective advantages and disadvantages. Some lead to more complications than others, including bleeding, crusting, breathing difficulties, scar tissue formation, dryness, and loss of nasal sensations. Technological developments in recent decades have led to the creation of improved surgical instruments that have made it easier and safer to cut smaller portions of turbinate tissue, resulting in fewer side effects. However, the possibility of complication remains. Any turbinate reduction procedure, if it involves removing too much healthy turbinate tissue or distorting too much of its form, can lead to ENS. As a rule, the more conservative the turbinate reduction technique, the less likely one is to develop serious complications such as ENS.

Turbinate Reduction Surgeries

+ submucous resection
+ submucous resection with outfracture
+ electrocautery
+ radiofrequency

> ## *Turbinate Reduction Surgeries (cont.)*
> ◆   total, subtotal and partial inferior turbinectomy
> ◆   other techniques:
>   –Injection corticosteroids
>   –Cryosurgery
>   –Laser surgery

Submucous Resection

Submucous resection is perhaps the safest turbinate surgery because of its diminished risk of bleeding and preservation of mucociliary clearance functioning.[1] A submucous resection procedure is used to either 1) remove part of the inferior turbinate bone while not tampering with overlying flaps of mucosa, or 2) remove vascular space tissue, which might be enlarged in patients with drug-induced rhinitis or sleep apnea. A small surgical blade, known as a microdebrider, is often used to extract precise amounts of tissue. An inferior turbinoplasty, a surgical technique Dr. Richard Mabry introduced, is similar to submucous resection as it involves removal of the turbinate bone, but also a posterior tip and a bit of the inferior turbinate mucosa are also cut.[2] These techniques are conservative because they leave much of the nasal mucosa untouched, although according to one study the results might be short-lived as the relapse rate was as high as 25%.[2] These procedures also involve greater manual dexterity than simple resection procedures.

Submucous Resection with Outfracture

Outfracture is a relatively safe turbinate surgery and it is often performed in conjunction with other turbinate surgeries, such as submucous resection and electrocautery. Outfracture literally means fracturing (breaking) the turbinate bone and then applying pressure on the bone to move it to the side or lateral wall of the nose. This procedure reduces the size and volume of the turbinate. The advantage of this procedure is the diminished risk of post-surgical complications such as bleeding or crusting. However, it might need to be repeated. Pontell, Slavit and Kern suggest outfracture is a relatively safe procedure, while Passali, Lauriello, Anselmi, and Bellussi recommend submucous resection with outfracture as one of the most effective turbinate surgeries with greatest preservation of nasal functioning. [3-4]

Electrocautery

One of the earliest types of turbinate surgery was electrocautery, introduced in 1845 by Heider from Vienna and Crusel from St. Petersburg.[5] A galvanic current would run through the turbinate with heat transforming turbinate tissue from liquid to solid. This caused necrosis (cell death) and ultimately shrank the turbinate. Because of the use of electrical currents and consequent necrosis, electrocautery has been criticized, particularly during the late 1800s and early 1900s.

New and improved methods of electrocautery have been introduced over the past century with major improvements in recent decades. One relatively new type of electrocautery procedure is submucosal diathermy, a type of electrocautery performed at lower temperatures beneath the mucous layer affecting areas of tissue where it is directly applied and having limited impact on neighboring turbinate tissue. While it is a relatively simple procedure to perform, it has been associated with crusting and regrowth of lesions.[6] Also, relief of nasal obstruction might be of a short duration, lasting months to years, and it might need to be repeated.[7]

Radiofrequency

Radiofrequency is a turbinate reduction procedure introduced in the 1990s that uses heat to induce submucosal tissue destruction. This procedure results in increased amounts of airflow through the nose and improvement in mucociliary clearance functioning with minimal complications. Only some mild swelling and rhinorrhea (runny nose) have been reported with radiofrequency techniques.[8] Specifically, coblation-assisted radiofrequency techniques help shrink tissue within the turbinates with high patient satisfaction and minimal complications.[9-10] However, coblation-assisted radiofrequency is not considered appropriate for people with enlarged bony turbinates. Radiofrequency is superior to electrocautery because the tissue temperatures, power levels, and voltage required are much lower, yet achieve the same result as electrocautery with less neighboring tissue damage.[11]

Total, Subtotal and Partial Inferior Turbinectomy

A turbinectomy, be it total, subtotal, or partial resection (the latter of which involves removing two-thirds of the turbinates) are methods still practiced today, although less commonly than in recent decades. But these procedures are controversial and their effects are *irreversible*. Additional turbinate tissue can always be trimmed later if necessary, but turbinate tissue cannot be recovered once too much is removed.

While Jones in 1895 and Holmes in 1900 advocated for total turbinectomies, this method was soon criticized for its irreversible effects. Speilberg, for example, warned of a doctor who might perform overly aggressive surgeries and not be content until every intranasal structure was removed.[12] Instead, Speilberg recommended submucous resection of the turbinates as a more conservative alternative. Because of adverse consequences reported from total and partial turbinectomies, similar to ENS symptoms, these procedures fell into disrepute from the early 1900s to the 1970s with more conservative turbinate reduction procedures preferred, such as submucous resection.

Remarkably, research articles in the 1970s and 1980s once again recommended total inferior turbinectomy, suggesting it had few side effects, which led to greater practice of it among ENTs and plastic surgeons.[13-17] These studies suggested total turbinectomies had little or no effect on dryness and crusting. According to Hol and Huizing, however, many of these research studies utilized past research that offered unproven opinions and did not include good outcome measures. For example, a study citing improvement from a total inferior turbinectomy might note the patient could smell better and has more air entering his or her nasal passages than before the turbinectomy, but it might not take into account subjective patient symptoms; objective measures, such as nasal patency—openness—do not necessarily correlate with patient symptoms.[9] A patient with ENS can have large, open nasal airways but feel as though he or she is not breathing adequately. Furthermore, most of these studies that examined aftereffects from turbinectomies did not track patient results for many years following surgery; for some ENS sufferers breathing problems might be detected early on after surgery, but significant dryness or mucosal atrophy might not develop until 8 or more years later.

During the 1980s and 1990s, an opposite, troubling explanation emerged: that symptoms of crusting, dryness and pain were prevalent in patients who underwent these procedures.[18-21] Specifically, the following has been reported about total inferior turbinectomies: post-operative hemorrhage rate of 10%; synechiae (scar tissue formation) 6-12% of the time; and nasal crusting, sometimes lasting for months, up to 15% at one year after surgery.[2] Partial turbinectomies, because they consist of less tissue removal than with total inferior turbinectomies, would likely have similar, but less severe, complications.

The landmark study "Atrophic Rhinitis: A Review of 242 Cases," by Drs. Moore and Kern, suggested a direct link between ENS and total and partial turbinectomies: of 157 patients with ENS, 110 underwent partial inferior and/or middle turbinectomies, and 47 had total removal of their middle and inferior turbinates.

Two classic research studies that compared how patients fared over several years with follow-up ratings of patient symptoms were completed by Moore, Freeman, Ogren, and Yonkers in 1985, and by Passali et al. in 1999. [4,18] Both articles cited post-operative problems associated with total inferior turbinectomies.

Moore et al. conducted a 3-5 year follow-up of 18 patients who received total inferior turbinectomies and found that 12 patients (66%) who underwent such procedures continued to experience chronic nasal crusting and an odor detectable by others, consistent with secondary atrophic rhinitis. Only 2 patients reported they were symptom-free. In other words, most patients in this study who underwent total inferior turbinectomy went on to develop serious problems, many of which were similar to ENS. Moore et al. argued that their study showed total inferior turbinectomies carry "significant morbidity and should be condemned."[22]

According to a research study conducted by Passali et al. that examined 6 different turbinate reduction procedures and followed-up on patients 4 years after surgery, total inferior turbinectomy had the most adverse affects of any turbinate surgery on nasal physiology. Patients who received total inferior turbinectomy had the poorest mucociliary transport time, the most dryness and crusting, and turbulent airflow into the nasal passages. It is clear that the more aggressive the surgery, the more complications might result. Dr. Kern's advice to colleagues: "Don't be a turbinator."[23]

Despite obvious concerns about complications of aggressive turbinate surgeries, a recent research study of 227 children under age 10 suggested that some children who suffer considerably from enlarged turbinates might actually benefit from total inferior turbinectomies, resulting in improved sleep and thinner nasal secretions.[24] Clearly, ENS awareness is needed!

In sum, a panel of experts from the American Rhinologic Society developed the following consensus statement on total inferior turbinectomies:

> *The excess removal of turbinate tissue might lead to empty nose syndrome. Excess resection can lead to crusting, bleeding, breathing difficulty [often the paradoxical sensation of obstruction], recurrent infections, nasal odor, pain, and often clinical depression. In one study, the mean onset of symptoms occurred more than 8 years following the turbinectomies.*[25]

Injection Corticosteroids

Injection of steroids is considered effective in reducing the size of an enlarged turbinate.[26] While a doctor can easily administer and it is cost-effective, steroids usually wear off after 6 weeks and a rare, but possible complication is blindness.[27]

Cryosurgery

Cryosurgery consists of freezing turbinate tissue and it is considered effective against controlling severe runny nose.[28] However, the amount of turbinate volume reduction is difficult to achieve and it can damage healthy nasal mucosa so results, when compared to other methods such as submucous resection, are disappointing. Consequently, it is not widely used today.

Laser Surgery

Laser surgery to treat enlarged turbinates was first used in the late 1970s.[29] This procedure consists of shooting a laser beam that is absorbed by the tissue, causing it to evaporate. However, this procedure has been associated with complications including destruction of nasal cilia, crusts, and formation of scar tissue.[30-31] Shooting a beam through the turbinate tissue would likely damage much healthy nasal mucosa in the process; furthermore, precise amount of tissue removal is arduous to achieve because of its reliance on a wavelength of light and the amount of energy applied. Unfortunately, this method that is heavily advertised in the daily newspaper can lead to ENS because excess mucosa is removed.

Middle Turbinate Resection

Much of the commentary in this section addresses reduction of the inferior turbinates rather than middle turbinates. More research has been done on inferior turbinate reduction procedures probably in part because inferior turbinates are much larger and their location in the nasal airway is more significant, as they process the majority of inspired air (causing more breathing problems than enlarged middle turbinates, although middle turbinates can also cause such difficulties). Unfortunately, total resection of the middle turbinate is considered in the standard range of nasal surgery today in part because the middle turbinates are smaller and play a less significant role in the airway, and complications from middle turbinate reduction procedures consequently seem fewer than with inferior turbinate reductions.[26, 32]

Middle turbinate resection procedures should only be performed as a last resort when there is ample reason, such as a significant polyp, a bent middle turbinate, or allergic fungal sinusitis. In conjunction with sinus surgery, part of the middle turbinate might be removed to access the ethmoid sinuses. Yet complete removal of the middle turbinate can cause significant scarring and obstruction of the frontal recess[t]. It can also contribute to differences in airway breathing, as well as sinus problems and over-sensitivity, because a normal middle turbinate hoods over the sinuses to protect them. Furthermore, this procedure can lead to a diminished sense of smell.

The Multiple Surgery Experience among ENS Patients

Many cases of ENS result from repeat surgeries as described in "Erasorama Surgery," an important research article by Drs. Mark May and Barry Shaitkin.[33] For example, the average number of surgeries among people who had turbinectomies (that later resulted in ENS) in Drs. Moore and Kern's study was 2.3.[34]

With the availability of the endoscope[u] to the American medical community in 1985, which enabled doctors to examine and operate upon nasal passages more conveniently than in the past, some doctors became more bold in their surgical approach.[25] This brazen mindset, combined with a lack of clear guidelines delineating a disorder to a particular

---

t *The frontal recess is the space between the frontal sinuses—the pair of sinus cavities in the forehead located above the eyes and behind the eyebrows—and groove in the lateral wall of the nasal cavity. Mucus from the frontal sinuses drains into the nose via the frontal recess.*

u *The Caldwell-Luc was commonly practiced in America until the 1980s when it was replaced by the endoscope, an improved technological tool consisting of a telescope attached to a video monitor. It is rarely practiced today but there are still some indications when it is necessary. Regrettably, it is also sometimes practiced today by surgeons who are not comfortable doing functional endoscopic sinus surgery. This procedure, also called traditional sinus surgery, consists of making an incision in the upper gums in order to either cut out inflamed sinus tissue or create a hole for mucus to drain.*

operation and no universally accepted standard for evaluating results of a surgery, has led to destructive consequences.

A hypothetical, although not necessarily common, overzealous series of surgeries might thus occur as follows: a patient with rhinitis presents with an unsuccessful history of medical treatment and can only describe what he or she feels in a few terms, such as "congested" or "stuffy."[33] A doctor might review the CT scan and notice anatomic abnormalities such as a mildly deviated septum and mucosal contact between the middle turbinate and septum (a normal anatomic variation). The patient is eager to undergo surgery to relieve him or her of his or her symptoms particularly because the surgery is low-risk.

The doctor performs a septoplasty and pares down part of the inferior and middle turbinates. This operation fails to clear up patient symptoms and the patient over time tries various remedies including nasal irrigation, nasal sprays and antibiotics. After one year has passed, the doctor then reviews the CT scan and notices even more inflamed tissue. The patient returns to the doctor and receives further surgery, including middle meatal antrostomies[v], an ethmoidectomy, and more middle and inferior turbinate reduction. As the condition worsens, the doctor searches for an explanation for these symptoms of obstruction, diminished sense of smell, and headaches, and blames the patient's original nasal problem (although the newfound symptoms are in large part a result of the turbinate surgery). The doctor then questions if not enough of the turbinates was removed during the first two operations.

In this example, such a doctor believes nasal obstruction is caused by an overly congested nose when the exact opposite is true: the obstruction

---

v *Middle meatal antrostomies consist of creating drainage holes from the middle meatus into the maxillary sinus.*

is occurring because the nose is too open! The end result of all these turbinate surgeries is an increasingly empty nose that is less functional.

This discussion of multiple surgeries is why a thorough discussion of what precisely will be done and how it will affect the mucosa of the turbinates must take place before any type of nasal surgery. Furthermore, advances brought about by improved surgical procedures are of little comfort to a patient whose breathing difficulties resulted from too much removal of turbinates. In this case, it is better to prevent the need for surgery in the first place!

My Ratings of Turbinate Surgeries

Key:
1=most effective at increasing nasal airway volume while preserving nasal mucosa
8=Least effective

Turbinate surgery	Rating	Comments
Submucous resection	2	Overall safe, conservative option
Submucous resection with outfracture	1	Safe and more effective than submucous resection alone
Electrocautery	4	Similar to radiofrequency, but perhaps not as effective; it burns and it is hard to determine depth
Radiofrequency	3	Positive results overall, but perhaps not as promising as once thought
Total inferior turbinectomy	8	Should be avoided at all costs
Partial turbinectomy	7	Relatively high risk of complications and it is irreversible
Injection corticosteroid	5	Limited duration of effectiveness
Laser surgery	6	Unwise, as it can damage outer mucosal layers

Future Thoughts on Turbinate Surgeries

Regardless of technique used, any surgery—even the best one—that consists of removing too much nasal mucosa can be harmful. A good question to ask is, "How much of the nasal mucosa, the organ of the nose, can one remove before contributing to ENS symptoms?" We just do not know. It appears that we can remove some of the turbinates and the nose works fine. But if too much tissue is removed, results are disastrous. In that sense it appears the more aggressive the turbinectomy, the greater the likelihood of ENS.

If you are considering turbinate surgery after less invasive interventions have been attempted (such as saline irrigation, allergy treatment, or antibiotics), you might wish to ask your doctor 3 questions so you can make an informed decision:

- What surgical procedure will be used?
- Which turbinates will be reduced?
- What percentage of the turbinates will be reduced? A higher percentage indicates a more aggressive surgery and greater risk of ENS.

If you have any doubt about possible surgery, obtain a second opinion. It might be the best decision you can make and could help put your mind at ease.

In closing, I offer the following thoughts on turbinate reduction procedures: if one is to undergo surgery, it is my hope doctors will choose conservative turbinate reduction operations and that patients will seek more conservative surgeries so that they will not end up with a complication as serious as ENS. You can always have more turbinate tissue removed later on, but you cannot recover it once too much is removed. While it is unfortunate that ENS is surgery-induced, it is reassuring that it can be largely eliminated in future generations if surgery is performed with greater caution. Fortunately, there appears to be an overall growing recognition among physicians that caution should be exercised when performing such a procedure.[35]

Chapter 5 References

1. Passali, D., Passali, F.M., Damiani, V., Passali, G.C., & Bellusi, L. (2005). Treatment of inferior turbinate hypertrophy: A randomized clinical trial. *Annals of Otology, Rhinology & Laryngology,* 112, 683-688.

2. Mabry, R.L. (1988). Inferior turbinoplasty: Patient selection, technique, and long-term consequences. *Otolaryngology - Head and Neck Surgery,* 98, 60.

3. Pontell, J., Slavit, D.H., & Kern, E.B. (1998). The role of outfracture in correcting post-rhinoplasty nasal obstruction. *Ear, Nose and Throat Journal,* 77, 106-108.

4. Passali, D., Lauriello, M., Anselmi, M., & Bellussi, L. (1999). Treatment of hypertrophy of the inferior turbinate: long-term results in 382 patients randomly assigned to therapy. *Annals of Otology, Rhinology & Laryngology,* 108, 569-575.

5. Hol, M.K., & Huizing, E.H. (2000). Treatment of inferior turbinate pathology: a review and critical evaluation of the different techniques. *Rhinology,* 38, 157-166.

6. Meredith, G.M., Jr. (1988). Surgical reduction of hypertrophied inferior turbinates: A comparison of electrofulguration and partial resection. *Plastic and Reconstructive Surgery,* 81, 891.

7. Goode, R.L., & Pribitkin, E. (1995). *Diagnosis and Treatment of Turbinate Dysfunction, 2nd Ed.* Alexandria: American Academy of Otolaryngology-Head and Neck Surgery, Inc., pp. 1-73.

8. Coste, A., Yona, L., Blumen, M., Louis, B., Zerah, F., Rugina, M., Peynegre, R., Harf, R., & Escudier, E. (2001). Radiofrequency is a safe and effective treatment of turbinate hypertrophy. *Laryngoscope,* 111, 894-899.

9. Bäck, LJJ, Hytönen, ML, Malmberg HO, & Ylikoski JS (2002). Submucosal bipolar radiofrequency thermal ablation of inferior turbinates: A long-term follow-up with subjective and objective assessment. *The Laryngoscope,* 112, 1806-1812.

10. Bhattacharyya, N., & Kepnes, L.J. (2003). Clinical effectiveness of coblation inferior turbinate reduction. *Otolaryngology - Head and Neck Surgery,* 129, 365-371.

11. Li, K.K., Powell, N.B., Riley, R.W., Troell, R.J., & Guilleminault, C. (1998). Radiofrequency volumetric tissue reduction for treatment of turbinate hypertrophy: a pilot study. *Otolaryngology - Head and Neck Surgery*, 119, 569-573.

12. Spielberg, W. (1924). The treatment of nasal obstruction by submucous resection of the inferior turbinate bone. *Laryngoscope*, 34, 197-203.

13. Fry, H.J.H. (1973). Judicious turbinectomy for nasal obstruction. *New Zealand Journal of Surgery*, 42, 291-294.

14. Courtiss, E.H., Goldwyn, R.M., Obrien, J.J. (1978). Resection of obstructing inferior turbinates. *Plastic and Reconstructive Surgery*, 62, 249-257.

15. Ophir, D., Shapira, A., & Marshank, G. (1985). Total inferior turbinectomy for nasal airway obstruction. *Archives of Otolaryngology*, 111, 93-95.

16. Odetoyinbo, O (1987). Complications following total inferior turbinectomy: facts or myths? *Archives of Otolaryngology*, 12, 361-363.

17. Thompson, A.C. (1989). Surgical reduction of the inferior turbinate in children: extended follow-up. *Journal of Laryngology and Otology*, 103, 577-579.

18. Moore, G.F., Freeman, T.J., Ogren, F.P., & Yonkers, A.J. (1985). Extended follow-up of total inferior turbinate resection for relief of chronic nasal obstruction. *Laryngoscope*, 95, 1095-1099.

19. Wight, R.G., Jones, A.S., & Beckham,E. (1990). Trimming of the inferior turbinates – a prospective, long-term study. *Clinical Otolaryngology and Allied Sciences*, 15, 247-350.

20. Salam, M.A. & Wengraf, C. (1993). Concho-antropexy or total inferior turbinectomy for hypertrophy of the inferior turbinates? *Journal of Laryngology and Otology*, 107, 1125-1128.

21. Carrie, S., Wright, R.G., Jones, A.S., Stevens, J.C., Parker, A.J. & Yardley, M.P.J, (1996). Long-term results of trimming of the inferior turbinates. *Clinical Otolaryngology and Allied Sciences*, 21, 139-141.

22. Moore, Freeman, Ogren, & Yonkers, 1985, P. 1099.

23. Kern, E.B. (2006, audioclip). *Click here to listen to Dr. Kern's ENS Lecture.* Retrieved November 24, 2006, from the Empty Nose Syndrome Association Web site: *www.emptynosesyndrome.org.*

24. Segal, S., Eviator, E., Berenholz, L., Kessler, A., & Shlamkovitch, N. (2003). Inferior turbinectomy in children. *American Journal of Rhinology*, 17, 69-74.

25. Rice, D.H., Kern, E.B., Marple, B.F., Mabry, R.L., & Friedman, W.H. (2003). The turbinates in nasal and sinus surgery: A consensus statement. *Ear, Nose and Throat Journal*, 73, 82-83. [P. 83].

26. Goode, R.L., & Pribitkin, E. (1995). *Diagnosis and Treatment of Turbinate Dysfunction, 2nd Ed.* Alexandria: American Academy of Otolaryngology-Head and Neck Surgery, Inc., pp. 1-73.

27. Mabry, R.L. (1981). Visual loss after intranasal corticosteroid injection: Incidence, causes, and prevention. *Archives of Otolaryngology*, 107, 481.

28. King, H.C. & Mabry, R.L. (1993). *A Practical Guide to the Management of Nasal and Sinus Disorders.* New York: Thieme Medical Publishers, Inc.

29. Lenz, H., Eichler, J., Schafer, G., & Salk, J. (1977). Parameters for argon laser surgery of the lower human turbinates: in vitro experiments. *Acta Otolaryngology*, 83, 360.

30. Fukutake, T., Yamashita, T, Tomoda, K., & Kumazawa, T. (1986). Laser surgery for allergic rhinitis. *Archives of Otolaryngology, Head and Neck Surgery*, 112, 1280-1282.

31. Kubota, I. (1995). Nasal function following carbon dioxide laser turbinate surgery for allergy. *American Journal of Rhinology*, 93, 155-161.

32. Houser, S.M. (2006c). Empty nose syndrome associated with middle turbinate resection. *Otolaryngology - Head and Neck Surgery*, 135, 972-973.

33. May, M., & Schaitkin, B.M. (2002). Erasorama surgery. *Current Opinion in Otolaryngology and Head and Neck Surgery*, 10, 19-21.

34. Moore, E.J., & Kern, E.B. (2001). Atrophic Rhinitis: A review of 242 cases. *American Journal of Rhinology*, 15, 355-361.

35. Metson, R., & Mardon, S. (2005). *The Harvard Medical Guide to Healing Your Sinuses.* New York, NY: McGraw-Hill.

Chapter Six

———— ⟨⟨⟨⟨⟩⟩⟩⟩ ————

Politics of Empty Nose

Too many ENT specialists and plastic surgeons display a lack of understanding regarding the etiology, symptoms, and treatments for ENS. Various factors that have contributed to this confusion include:

1) Some doctors remain stuck on deceiving logic.
2) Logic leads some to believe removing even more turbinate tissue is best.
3) ENTs and plastic surgeons notice positive benefits to some patients.
4) ENS is less likely to be identified because of its iatrogenic origin.
5) Doctors (mistakenly) consider ENS rare.
6) Turbinate surgeries are financially 'sanctioned.'
7) There is a failure to adequately address ENS.

While ENT specialists have become increasingly aware in recent years that turbinate surgeries should be performed conservatively, it takes time for new ideas to become accepted into the mainstream, which means some ENTs are more cautious than others and some nasal surgeries do still result in ENS. Fortunately, it is likely fewer nasal surgeries result in ENS than 10 years ago.

A *New York Times* reporter writing for the *Milwaukee Journal Sentinel*, Gabrielle Glaser, touched upon this increasingly cautious attitude in a 2003 article, "For Chronic Sinusitis, Some Doctors Start Over."[1] This article asserted doctors in recent decades have been more aggressive in their attempts to remove turbinates, but are now learning the latter might have created more problems than it solved.

You might be questioning at this point, "If doctors are overall more conservative today than 10 years ago, do turbinate surgeries still lead to ENS?" Absolutely—if you are considering turbinate surgery, you are at risk for ENS! While the days of radical, total inferior turbinectomies are largely over, patients whose turbinate surgeries led to ENS in recent years would certainly affirm this risk. Some ENS sufferers are reporting severe breathing difficulties from surgeries done within the past year—and their doctors don't believe them!

Some Doctors Remain Stuck on Deceiving Logic

Simple logic partly accounts for confusion of ENS. If an artery is blocked, you unblock it by removing the clot. If the nose is blocked by an enlarged turbinate, you unblock it by taking it out. Makes sense. But the science of turbinates suggests this line of reasoning is incorrect.

The primary turbinates, after all, are similar in size to a finger, incredibly complex, serve many important functions in the nose and they should be treated with utmost respect like other important body parts such as a toe. If you have a swollen toe, do you try to treat it first or cut it off? And if you cut it off, do you expect the foot to be fully functional? No, it's partly amputated because the area where the toe used to be is now empty. So is the nose after the turbinates have been removed.

Logic Leads Some to Believe Removing
Even More Turbinate Tissue is Best

Unfortunately, this logic has led some doctors to believe that more turbinate tissue removal leading to increased airflow through the nose equals good results. If these doctors believe that, they are not likely to recognize ENS as a serious problem. Rather, they will perceive an increasingly empty nose as acceptable with presumed benefits to the patient.

In 2004, at the prestigious American Academy of Otolaryngology conference, for instance, a prominent ENT surgeon lectured that removing turbinates is good medicine and he will often remove more turbinate tissue if the patient still reports blockage.[2] He claimed there were no complications!

ENTs and Plastic Surgeons Notice Positive Benefits to Some Patients

The fact that some, but not all, turbinate reduction surgeries result in ENS means they will continue to be performed. If turbinate reduction surgeries always resulted in ENS symptoms, they would have ended long ago. A doctor might thus observe his or her other patients were helped by a similar procedure, and when the patient is still symptomatic 3 months later, they are perplexed by the symptoms and the radiologist reports sinusitis instead of ENS. Radiologists will not mention excess space as a disease.

ENS Less Likely to be Identified Because of its Iatrogenic Origin

In addition, when a problem is "created" by a doctor via surgery, the natural inclination is not to acknowledge it or actively deny it is real. It would be a self-indictment for a doctor to admit he or she has created such a significant problem.

If ENS was caused by genetic factors, I surmise it would be taken much more seriously by the medical community and would have already received proper medical attention. Consider Sjogren's syndrome, which has genetic, hormonal and immunologic causes. This syndrome is an autoimmune disease where the body's immune system mistakenly attacks its own moisture-producing glands; dry mouth and eyes are its 2 common symptoms, and it has about 4,000,000 sufferers in America. This condition has received attention and proper recognition, but ENS, which has severe symptoms in its own right, has not.

Doctors (Mistakenly) Consider ENS Rare

Some ENT doctors might assume that empty nose is rare since they do not encounter it often. Yet even if most turbinate reduction procedures do not result in ENS, there still remains the possibility that millions of Americans are suffering from it. The National Center for Health Statistics (NCHS), which is a branch of the Centers for Disease Control and Prevention (CDC), last reported turbinectomy and nasal surgery rates in 1996, but has not produced surveys since due to a lack of funding.[3] During 1996, the NCHS reported that 161,000 turbinectomies were performed.[4] A turbinectomy, in this definition, ranges from a conservative technique that spares healthy nasal tissue and involves removal of less than 33% of a turbinate to a more aggressive operation that involves removal of 70-100% of a turbinate. The 161,000 turbinectomies excluded ambulatory surgery patients who were admitted to hospitals as inpatients; it only refers to outpatient surgeries, which happens more often with conservative procedures, whereas radical turbinectomies frequently require at least one day of hospitalization. Furthermore, turbinectomies are often done as a secondary procedure at the same time as another operation. For example, many people with ENS have undergone multiple procedures, such as functional endoscopic sinus surgery (FESS) and/or a septoplasty, with the turbinate surgery as a secondary procedure. In addition, doctors will often cut at least a portion of the middle turbinates to reach certain sections of the nose, such as the ethmoid sinuses. Such procedures might only officially register as one septoplasty, although turbinates were also reduced in size during the operation. Therefore, besides the certain 161,000 turbinectomies, there were also 2,091,000 operations on the "nose, mouth, and pharynx," and 276,000 operations of "repair and plastic operations on the nose."[4] That is a total of 2,528,000 operations that might involve a turbinate reduction procedure in the United States in 1996 alone.

My estimate that at least 500,000 turbinate reduction procedures are performed per year in the United States represents a reasonable estimate. If only 20% of such procedures results in ENS symptoms, that means there are 100,000 new cases of ENS per year in the United States. Over 20 years that amounts to 2,000,000 ENS sufferers in the United States—and counting[w].

Perhaps the most accurate way, however, to discover the incidence of ENS would be to look at microstatistics, not macrostatistics. Microstatistics might consist of reviewing all the cases of one doctor who performed turbinate reduction procedures, following these patients for at least 10 years, and then contacting them for updated information. Exams would consist of pre- and post-surgery measures with a valid measure of patient symptoms. Although a difficult task, it would be helpful and enlightening for a doctor to pursue this line of research, and the possible rate of ENS in the population could then be generalized. Until then the actual incidence of ENS remains unknown and all aforementioned commentary is merely speculation.

---

w Given significant diagnostic confusion, I believe the number of ENS sufferers in the United States might be even much higher than 2 million. I question if many ENS sufferers are simply unaware that they, in fact, have ENS. Furthermore, keep in mind that the United States' population is only 5% of the world's population, so the number of ENS sufferers worldwide could represent 20 times the number of sufferers in the U.S., assuming a constant rate of turbinate surgeries between countries.

Finally, consider the following admissions from two well-respected doctors. Dr. Houser reports seeing new empty nose CT scans once per week, while Dr. Patricia Hudgins, a neuroradiologist with specialty in head and neck radiology from Emory University in Atlanta, Georgia, reports seeing such CT scans at least several times per week.[5-6] Because Dr. Hudgins treats complex cases and her field of specialty is neuroradiology, her report might be an overestimate of the incidence as a whole.[7] Nevertheless, she noted that all of her patients with empty nose scans have undergone a septoplasty, and that all have some portion of their middle and/or inferior turbinates missing. Interestingly, she suggested ENS appears to be a frequent problem among patients who reported "chronic sinus symptoms." She and Dr. Houser believe the incidence of ENS is higher than assumed and it is underreported in the medical literature.

Turbinate Surgeries are Financially 'Sanctioned'

Regrettably, insurance companies actually encourage turbinectomy procedures![2] Doctors must adhere to following rigid CPT codes when performing procedures, otherwise insurance companies—which make the rules and pay the fees—will not recognize the procedure. They list turbinectomy as one of the accepted procedures for which they will pay. This puts forth the suggestion that turbinectomy is an "approved" and "honored" procedure rather than a special procedure that can spare healthy nasal mucosa. Since it is approved and sanctioned, a doctor might reasonably conclude they should do this procedure to open up the airway.

Failure to Adequately Address ENS

ENS has been underreported in medical literature, which makes it appear that ENT doctors and plastic surgeons are reluctant to address this problem. Someone researching ENS will discover there are not many journal articles that specifically deal with ENS. I can only think of two offhand—"Atrophic Rhinitis: A Review of 242 Cases" by Moore and Kern, and "Empty Nose Syndrome Associated with Middle Turbinate Resection" by Houser—that is it. Also consider that according to Dr. Grossan, when the concept of ENS was presented at the Triologic meeting about 5 years ago, the response was reported to be a deafening silence.[8] The response at the 2006 annual convention of the American Rhinologic Society was even worse: there was not a single presentation on ENS.

The end result of these politics is that if ENS continues to be largely ignored by ENTs and plastic surgeons, innocent patients will continue to be afflicted with this terrible complication of nasal surgery and veteran ENS sufferers will continue to remain largely untreated and ignored by medical professionals. We cannot let that happen.

Chapter 6 References

1. Glaser, G. (2003, Jan. 6). *For chronic sinusitis, some doctors start over.* Retrieved December 16, 2006 from Find Articles Web site at: *www.calbears.findarticles.com/p/articles/mi_qn4196/is_20030106/ai_n10858608.* [Para. 18].

2. Grossan, M. (personal communication, March 25, 2007).

3. Chase, J.M. (personal communication, November 20, 2006).

4. Department of Health and Human Services, Center for Disease Control and Prevention (2006). *Advance Data from Vital and Health Statistics, No. 300.* Retrieved November 24, 2006, from the Web site: *www.cdc.gov/nchs/data/ad/ad300t4.pdf* [P. 1].

5. Houser, S.M. (personal communication, January 26, 2007).

6. Hudgins, P.A. (personal communication, January 24, 2007).

7. Hudgins, P.A. (personal Communication, January 26, 2007).

8. Grossan, M. (personal communication, January 19, 2007).

Chapter Seven

ENS: *The Difficult Diagnosis*

There are numerous reasons ENS is difficult to diagnose. As noted, there is much confusion that exists in the medical literature on the etiology, symptoms and treatment of it. Doctors respect peer-reviewed research that discusses a medical condition but, with exceptions mentioned, there is a lack of research on ENS. Consequently, ENS seems poorly understood at best, highly overlooked at worst.

Below are 5 factors contributing to diagnostic confusion of ENS:

1. There is a lack of knowledge on ENS among ENTs and Plastic Surgeons.
2. There is no objective test to determine ENS.
3. The ENS patient is in denial of his or her symptoms.
4. The suffering experienced by the patient is in relation to how he or she felt before surgery.
5. Severe dryness and atrophy might not occur until years after surgery.

There is a Lack of Knowledge on ENS among ENTs and Plastic Surgeons

In most professions you are likely to practice what you are taught, and ENT doctors and plastic surgeons are no exception. It takes a while for new ideas and treatments to become mainstreamed in and for doctors to adopt new practices. ENT doctors and plastic surgeons trained during the 1970s and 1980s, for example, are more apt to believe that a total inferior turbinectomy is safe because literature of that time advocated for this procedure, while doctors trained in more recent years might believe turbinate surgeries should be performed more cautiously due to a growing awareness of complications of these surgeries.

Furthermore, most doctors have not personally had ENS so they would not know how to cope with it, while others might not evaluate the "whole" patient. For example, a patient might have allergies, which are left untreated and are causing enlarged turbinates and ultimately leading to frequent sinus infections. Rather than treat allergies through allergy injections or sinus infections through saline irrigation, some doctors might suggest cutting more turbinate tissue since the inferior turbinates are blocking breathing. Or, if after allergy treatment the turbinates continue to block breathing, the allergist might refer the patient to an ENT for a surgical solution.

While current understanding is that the entire upper and lower respiratory tract is one organ, ENT doctors and plastic surgeons might not be aware of the effect of loss of nasal airflow resistance on lung functioning, as a pulmonologist (lung doctor) would. They might note the nose provides 50% of the nasal resistance that is vital for lung functioning, but not be sure why it is vital. For example, Dr. Pat Barelli argued that doctors have largely ignored the role of nasopulmonary activity and specifically the role of the nose in respiration, despite more than a hundred years of medical literature and clinical experience in these areas.[1] Consequently, a doctor might recognize that an aggressive turbinate surgery might result in disorderly incoming nasal airflow that does not ventilate all areas of the nose, but not necessarily recognize that too low of nasal resistance leads to inefficient gas-exchange in the alveoli of the lungs that manifests itself as micro-areas of poor lung ventilation.

There is No Objective Test to Determine ENS

There is no objective test to confirm ENS is present in a patient, although this is also true of other disorders of the ear, nose and throat. Objective means it can be verified by physical evidence (such as a thermometer measuring one's temperature), while subjective implies personal interpretation that is not readily observable. One disorder that relies on a subjective report of symptoms is tinnitus, which consists of a perception of ringing or buzzing in the ears or head, despite no actual origin of the noise. With ENS, CT scans will show empty space but not the patient's sensation of "not getting enough air." A doctor must therefore rely on a patient's subjective complaint of symptoms, such as reporting of disturbed nasal breathing. ENT doctors, however, are primarily trained to look for physical signs of dryness, crusting, fetor, or atrophy after turbinate surgeries, and they might consequently disregard subjective complaints that occur more frequently after these surgeries—complaints that indicate ENS symptoms. While subjective, the symptoms of ENS are indeed real and do stem from a physical origin.

Papay, Eliachar, and Risica argue, for example, that a *common* complication after an overly aggressive turbinate surgery is rhinitis sicca, which includes inadequate nasal humidification.[2] As stated in chapter 4, ENS in some cases is similar or tantamount to rhinitis sicca. So perhaps the likelihood of developing ENS after an overly aggressive turbinate surgery is much higher than previously thought or reported in the medical literature.

The ENS Patient is in Denial of His or Her Problem

The patient also plays a role in diagnosis. Many patients who experience ENS symptoms shortly after surgery will remain in denial of them for a number of reasons:

◆ The actual physiology behind ENS is confusing and most patients will not intuitively understand it. For instance, they will not identify why they are short or breath or why their sleep seems shallow. They might fully blame other conditions such as hypertension, diabetes, sleep apnea, or obesity, rather than the turbinate resection itself for their breathing or sleeping problems.

◆ Some ENS patients who suffered tremendously from years of chronic nasal obstruction associated with rhinitis will experience temporary relief of having an "open nose."

◆ ENS patients have a very difficult time accepting that they underwent an elective procedure, such as a turbinate reduction surgery, and might blame themselves that they did not do enough research beforehand.

◆ Many patients are apt to return to the doctor who caused ENS, rather than seeking another doctor who might, perhaps, provide a more objective opinion on their medical condition. Consequently, they believe what they are told by their doctor.

◆ The ENS patient might have trusted his or her doctor, which can make it very hard to accept that the doctor might have caused a significant problem.

The Suffering Experienced by the Patient is in Relation to How He or She Felt Before the Turbinate Surgery

Many people with ENS go from feeling their airways are too closed before surgery to too open after, and some patients feel relief that can last for a while. That alone makes it more difficult for patients to identify ENS as a "problem." Many patients might perceive that their nasal passages are more open prior to surgery and deem their post-surgical state as improved, even though the ensuing breathing is much more problematic than they think. If they believe they have a problem after surgery, they might simply blame the original condition (before surgery).

Severe Dryness and Atrophy Might Not Occur Until Years After Surgery

The patient might not recognize ENS symptoms immediately, particularly if he or she has enjoyed at least some relief, or because the nose is healing after an operation and it has to completely drain blood clots and crusts, which might take weeks or even months. Yet it can take years for severe dryness to occur and for it to result in atrophy of the nasal mucosa. Years after surgery many patients might not connect their current symptoms with their operation years earlier, and doctors, for their own self-interests, might not encourage them to connect the two.

Chapter 7 References

1. Beverly H. Timmons & Ronald Ley, Eds. (1994). *Behavioral and Psychological Approaches to Breathing Disorders.* New York: Plenum Press. [Section, 47-58, by Dr. Pat Barelli].

2. Papay, F.A., Eliachar, I., & Risica, R. (1991). Fibromuscular temporalis graft implantation for rhinitis sicca. *Ear, Nose and Throat Journal, 70,* 381-384.

Chapter Eight

What ENS Is Not: Postnasal Drip

A case example of someone with postnasal drip (PND) is as follows:

"Joe," age 39, is athletic, eats right and exercises. He has about one minor cold a year. Three years ago he had a bad sinus infection, but it cleared with medication. He complains because he feels a constant drainage of thick mucus in the back of his throat and his throat frequently feels sore, but not bad enough to see a doctor.

Finally Joe saw a doctor last month, took 4 weeks of amoxicillin, and his throat is essentially the same, although he has less nasal drainage. Upon examination Joe shows a mild redness in his nose. He has "bumps" or "lines" on the back of his throat in areas where lymphocytes have gathered together to fight infection. This is called posterior lymphoid hyperplasia. He then used pulsatile nasal and throat irrigation and drank many cups of hot tea, which in turn stimulated the body's natural healing elements and the "bumps" went away.

While the nose produces 1-2 liters of mucus per day that is swept into the pharynx and swallowed without notice, PND is a sensation of thick mucus in the back of one's nose where drainage in the throat can be felt. In the case of PND, the cilia slow down and do not help sweep the mucus blanket properly.

PND is noticed under 2 circumstances:

1) Various inflammatory responses including vasomotor rhinitis, allergic rhinitis, a sinus infection, or the common cold.

2) Mucosal dryness as a result of medications, a dry environment, dehydration, or mucosal thinning or loss.

Mucus production helps the nasal cilia move and acts as a canal to bring good white cells to where they may be needed to attack bacteria. If the cilia slow down, however, the mucus remains in place instead of being swept to the back of the throat and disposed of in the stomach. Consequently, the throat may become quite dry because nasal mucus is not moistening it, significantly affecting the voice. As cilia sweep the mucus, this mucus may also enter the throat under the mucous membrane in which case there are throat symptoms of pain and "something stuck in my throat."

One condition that leads to PND is vasomotor rhinitis, the primary symptom of which is a runny nose. Here the nerves of the nose that increase secretions are very active and there is a steady stream of thin mucus. Since it is a nerve stimulation issue, it does not respond to allergy treatment. There is a medication called Atrovent® that effectively treats this condition because it is a nerve blocker.

Allergies can also cause an excess amount of mucus to form and give PND symptoms. Usually the mucus is thin and not especially symptomatic. A patient may insist on blowing and sniffing as hard as possible, but doing so irritates the nose and causes an increase in mucus production. Conversely, allergy pills, Astelin® spray, or allergy shots may solve the problem.

In the acute stage of allergy, when the season starts, the nose runs freely and there is no infection. But in the late stage of allergy when the patient has been sneezing non-stop for 6 weeks and the nasal cilia are exhausted, then infection can set in. A sinus infection can follow a bad allergy, but allergy is not the cause of a sinus infection.

Tips to Prevent a Sinus Infection in the Late Stage of Allergy

- Use nose and throat pulsatile irrigation
- Drink hot tea
- Eat chicken soup
- Take mucus-thinners
- Take nasal steroid sprays
- Use vaporizers
- Take oral decongestants

ENS Versus PND

ENS	PND
Nose is dry	Nose may be moist
Mucus is thick and sticky	Mucus is liquid
Some nasal crusting	No crusting
Dry, irritated feeling in the throat	Throat tickled, but moist
May be improved but not cured	Cleared in 2 weeks by pulsatile irrigation
Often has diminished sense of smell	Can smell fine

Normal mucus may also become thick due to dryness caused by medications such as antihistamines, a dry environment, dehydration, or mucosal thinning or loss. In these instances the patient is aware of a ropy, thick material in the back of the throat affecting the voice.

Whether it is ENS or PND, you can acquire "new tissue" on the back of your throat. These essentially are and look like tonsil tissue under a microscope. The back of the throat can grow tonsil tissue that is essentially a clump of lymphoid (white cells) that are concentrated to filter out bacteria. The more bacteria come from the nose, the more lymphoid hyperplasia. It is important to know that this is not a cancer or "growth," but a normal response to excess bacteria.

As a rule, PND is not a serious condition unless it results in chest symptoms. Drainage from the nose can appear in and affect the chest in 16 hours. So if PND is annoying and there is an associated chest problem, a doctor must examine you promptly. The condition might be COPD, bronchitis, or asthma.

Tips for Treating PND

- Saline nasal spray
- Nasal gel
- Pulsatile throat irrigation (to increase circulation to area)
- Chicken soup
- Menthol lozenges
- Evaluation by an ENT to better define the problem and offer more specific answers

---

What Postnasal Drip is Not: GERD

Sometimes patients will experience an issue directly within their throat that they will perceive as PND, but it is actually gastroesophagael reflux disease (GERD), also known as acid reflux (although it may also be tonsillitis or a swallowing disorder). GERD is a condition that results from acid in the stomach flowing upward rather than downward.

A case example of someone with GERD is as follows:

"Jane," age 23, was a vocal performance student who lost her fine singing voice. She gargled regularly but that did not help. Her doctor tried antibiotics but that did not seem to help either. She saw an ENT doctor who looked at her nose and sinuses with an endoscope and declared the nose normal. He looked at her larynx (voicebox) with an instrument called a flexible laryngoscope. He saw that the vocal cords were normal but the back of the larynx, where it meets the front of the esophagus, was red and swollen. This area is called the arytenoids, and the inter-arytenoid tissue on the posterior side showed inflammation. This is what was impairing her voice.

When the doctor sees the part where acid from the stomach was irritating the voice box, he can make a correct diagnosis of GERD. She was treated with instructions and an acid inhibitor.

Singers are particularly prone to getting GERD because they put a lot of pressure on their stomach when singing. They eat very light before a performance, but too much before going to bed. Their stomach is still digesting the food so acid gets into the throat.

GERD may lead to a constant sore throat even when there is no history of indigestion. The ENT doctor can make the diagnosis by physical examination. The family doctor may try acid inhibitors such as Nexium® or Axid®. Other diagnostic methods include looking at the esophagus with an instrument—esophagoscopy—or putting a string down that measures the acid of that area.

Furthermore, GERD, PND, or asthma can all lead to a chronic cough, and treatment of the source of the cough will be most effective in eliminating it. The source of a cough for many ENS sufferers is thick mucus in the back of the nose and upper throat, which causes a gag reflex. This reflex, in turn, causes them to cough and it can lead to acid reflux. It is thus important for ENS sufferers to attempt to put mind over matter by clearing the throat lightly rather than forcefully, so as to prevent stomach acid from flowing upward. The more frequently and harder an ENS sufferer coughs, the more acid reflux he or she will have. Conversely, the more an ENS sufferer follows treatment strategies for PND and those outlined in chapter 9, particularly strategies in accordance with Principle 1, "Keep the nose moist while keeping mucus moving," the less reflux he or she will have.

Tips for Treating GERD

- Avoid caffeine and alcohol
- Avoid spices
- Eat smaller meals
- Lose weight
- Don't eat after 8 PM
- Elevate the head of the bed about 8 inches
- Take antacids

Chapter Nine

———— ⬡ ————

Non-Surgical Treatments for Empty Nose Syndrome

The following discussion regarding non-surgical treatments for ENS is based partly on my experiences and those of other empty nose sufferers. The ideas for intervention are not exhaustive; they do not cover every treatment that can be helpful for ENS, but outlines what I believe constitute the most important ones. As stated in the disclaimer, the treatments discussed do not constitute medical advice and I strongly recommend you discuss treatment strategies with your doctor prior to attempting any of the ones recommended here. I take no responsibility for decisions made based upon the following discussion; always seek professional medical advice. Seeking help from your medical doctor on a regular basis is one of the best courses of action you can take so any issues that arise can be promptly addressed, properly diagnosed, and effectively treated.

What to do if you Suspect Empty Nose

If you suspect possible ENS immediately following a turbinate reduction procedure, do not panic because you might not have it. Although ENS symptoms can in fact be experienced shortly after turbinate surgery, the symptoms you are experiencing might simply represent a temporary complication of nasal surgery. Congestion, dryness, crusting and bleeding, to name a few, are commonly experienced after surgery. If you experience these symptoms, consult with your doctor immediately and follow your doctor's recommendations for your particular situation.

If, however, an extended period of time such as 6 months passes and you are still experiencing symptoms that you believe might resemble ENS, you might consider asking your doctor to refer you for a follow-up CT scan. You could then discuss this scan with your doctor and ask which turbinates and what percentage of these turbinates were removed. Your doctor can also lead you to proper treatments. Should your doctor not be familiar with ENS, you might seek help from a doctor who is more experienced with ENS. You might also seek another source of information on ENS, such as Dr. Houser's website, *www.geocities.com/ shouser144/index.html.* If you do seek a second opinion, it is important your doctors communicate with each other, which will lead to a better diagnosis and improved outcome.

Three Guiding Principles for Good Nasal Health

Principle 1: Keep the nose moist while keeping mucus moving

Principle 2: Maintain blood supply to the nose by stimulating remaining turbinate tissue

Principle 3: Relax

The 3 guiding principles for good nasal health include keeping the nose moist, maintaining good blood supply to the nose, and ensuring plenty of relaxation. People suffering from other sinus problems, such as sinusitis, allergic rhinitis, and postnasal drip can also use some of these treatment strategies as many of the treatment principles apply in maintaining nasal and sinus health for all conditions. Use of these treatment strategies might, in fact, help prevent the need for surgery and result in improved nasal health for those who do not have ENS.

Keeping the nose moist is important to enhance mucociliary clearance system functioning. This principle is particularly important for the ENS sufferer because excessive dryness over time, as with an ENS nose, can ultimately lead to metaplasia, or total dysfunction, of the mucous membrane. Keeping mucus moving can be done in various ways including washing away bacteria, viruses, mold and fungi, thinning mucus, reducing inflammation, and constricting blood vessels (as with a decongestant). The treatment strategies in Principle 1 are broken down into natural, medical, dietary, and environmental remedies.

Principle 2 is keeping good blood supply to the nose, which is important to ensure improvement of nasal sensations. The nose is like a muscle; you use it more, it strengthens, but if you don't use it, it weakens. People with ENS report feeling much improvement in their nasal sensations after doing activities that lead to increased blood flow to the nose.

Principle 3 is to simply relax. The parasympathetic nervous system is closely connected to the nose. Relaxation techniques promote healing by stimulating the body's natural elements to fight infection.

2-Step Approach

With these 3 principles in mind, I recommend a simple 2-step approach for taking control of your nasal health:

1) Seek to incorporate 1-2 treatments from each of Principles 1, 2 and 3 in your daily routine. That is a total of 3-6 treatments per day. You might write down specifically what you are going to do, which will encourage and remind you to actually do it. You should also prioritize what is most important. An example treatment plan might be doing pulsatile irrigation 2 times per day, drinking eight 8-ounce glasses of water per day, exercising 3 times per week, and sleeping 8 hours per night. Of course you can do

as many treatments as you wish, but you should stick to what you know you can do faithfully; otherwise you will lose track and not do it. Remember, you will need to talk with your doctor about these treatments before attempting them. Your doctor must be a key player in helping you diagnose your specific medical problem and he or she might recommend or prescribe medications or other treatments.

2) If you are diagnosed with ENS and these treatments have not improved your breathing difficulties, you should talk with your ENT specialist who can help determine if you are a candidate for implant surgery or make a referral.

Principle 1: Keep the Nose Moist While Keeping Mucus Moving

Key Strategies

Natural remedies

+ Saline irrigation
+ Nasal sprays
+ Nasal gels
+ Nasal oils

Medical remedies

+ Irrigation with antibiotics
+ Guaifenesin
+ Zinc lozenges
+ Allergy shots
+ Antihistamines
+ Three vaccines
+ Decongestants
+ Anti-inflammatories

Principle 1: Keep the Nose Moist
While Keeping Mucus Moving (cont.)

Dietary remedies

- ✦ Plenty of fluids
- ✦ Hot tea with lemon and honey
- ✦ Chicken soup
- ✦ Vitamins (particularly A and D)
- ✦ Dietary considerations

Environmental remedies

- ✦ Environmental considerations
- ✦ Humidifier
- ✦ Good hygiene

NATURAL REMEDIES

Saline Irrigation

A very important principle for me in treating ENS is to ensure I keep my nose moist at all times through saline irrigation, which takes only a few minutes in the morning and evening. I believe this treatment can also be tremendously effective and should be the number one treatment for people suffering from sinuses, allergies and postnasal drip. *I wish saline irrigation was as well understood for treating the nose as washing hands is for cleaning dirty hands.*

ENS sufferers have chronically dry noses and dryness can lead to diminished cilia functioning. Consequently, they will have difficulty removing bacteria, viruses, mold, or fungi that enter their sinuses unless they literally wash them out. That is why nasal irrigation is so important and preventative. For ENS sufferers it might represent the *only way* to expel such particles that might otherwise remain stagnant in the mucus and lead to frequent infections.

By 2001, Dr. Grossan estimated 10% (or 40,000) purchasers of his Hydro Pulse® Irrigator were ENS sufferers based upon interviews and feedback.[1]

I use pulsatile saline irrigation about two times per day, and I would highly recommend rinsing out both your nose and throat each time you use it. It is helpful to rinse out the throat because it often contains phlegm (thick, sticky mucus) that has accumulated. Remember, it is important to keep mucus moving.

While various methods of nasal irrigation have been introduced, such as using a rubber bulb syringe (inside of the bulb can house bacteria), a neti pot, or a lavage bottle, I prefer the Grossan Hydro Pulse® Nasal-Sinus Irrigation System[x] as the best method for treating ENS (and other conditions) for 3 reasons:

1. It pulses at a rate to stimulate cilia to their best rhythm (16 pulses per second), helping to restore cilia functioning whereas other methods of saline irrigation do not.

2. It allows the user to irrigate *both* the nose and throat. I find it important to irrigate my throat regularly to bring circulation to the throat, thereby thinning mucus and reducing postnasal drip.

3. It can literally "wash away" allergic rhinitis. One study showed that people with allergies to pollen who used pulsatile irrigation regularly were able to significantly reduce the levels of IgE in the nose and bloodstream with reduced inflammation of the nasal mucosa.[2] Some of these patients even stopped taking allergy medication!

---

x *You can purchase Dr. Grossan's products, including the Hydro Pulse® Irrigator, through his commercial website at www.hydromedonline.com.*

A saline solution contains salt and water. The solution should be isotonic (meaning it has the same ratio of salt that is in your body) so it does not irritate your nasal passages. The mixture might be hypertonic (more salt per solution than in the body), which is helpful if the sinus membranes are swollen and hold more fluid; the belief is that salt will draw out the fluid. Too much of a hypertonic mixture, however, might lead to increased dryness in an already dry, empty nose.

Breathe-ease® XL Nasal Moisturizer Irrigation Solution (from Hydro Med Inc.) has been my choice to use when irrigating my nose because it is preservative-free and soothing on my sinuses. It contains many of the body's natural salts, including calcium chloride, potassium chloride, sodium chloride, and xylitol (a sugar that may help keep bacteria and fungi from adhering to the mucosal lining).

If you choose to make your own isotonic saline solution, purchase baking soda and either Kosher or pickling salt (salts that do not contain any preservatives, such as benzalkonium chloride, mercury, silica, or iodine). Preservatives must be avoided because they can lead to irritation of delicate nasal tissue if frequently applied. Add 1 teaspoon of salt to 16 ounces (500 ml) of lukewarm water. Then add half as much baking soda to reduce the stinging sensation from the salt (some ENS sufferers believe in adding just as much baking soda as salt to further reduce or eliminate the stinging sensation). You can also pre-mix the baking soda and salt before putting it into the water.

Preservatives to Avoid in Saline Solution

1. Benzalkonium chloride
2. Mercury
3. Silica
4. Iodine

How to Irrigate with the Grossan Hydro Pulse®

First you might heat water in the microwave so it is at least lukewarm. Then, in accordance with instructions, add 1 full teaspoon of Breathe-ease® solution or your own devised saline solution to 500 ml of water. Next, put these ingredients in your Grossan Hydro Pulse® Irrigator and bend your head (not turned to the side) over the sink. You should make a stream 1 inch high and, with the nasal pick inserted by the tip of your nose, aim the stream toward the sinus openings rather than the lateral wall or septum. You might wish to irrigate both nostrils with 250 ml so each side is equally cleansed. For throat irrigation, preparations are the same, but place the throat tip toward the back of the tongue and irrigate both sides with 250 ml. Also, please note you will need to follow the directions for weekly cleaning of the Hydro Pulse® Irrigator.

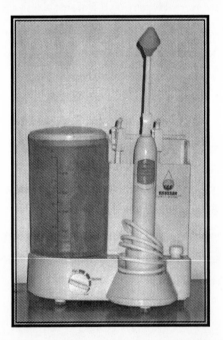

Figure 12. The Grossan Hydro Pulse®

Nasal Sprays

Frequent nasal sprayings is an important mechanism for irrigating my nose throughout the day, and it can be helpful for all sinus sufferers. Nasal sprays provide a quick, easy way to improve moisture content in the nose, thin mucus, and they can be used as often as needed. It has become part of my routine in treating ENS, as I keep a nasal spray in my pocket at all times. I probably spray my nose about every hour. The same principle applies to nasal sprays as in saline irrigation: make absolutely certain to use a spray that contains no harmful preservatives, such as benzalkonium chloride.

I believe use of Breathe-ease® XL Nasal Moisturizer Irrigation Solution with an accompanying 1 ounce refillable spray bottle is an economical, comfortable way to keep the nose moist. To create the mixture for the spray add ¼ teaspoon of Breathe-ease® XL solution to 4 ounces of water, mix, put the mixture in the spray bottle, then spray away! Just one refillable spray bottle of Breathe-ease® XL can last for more than 80 weeks. However, it is important to change the bottle's contents at least every 7 days because Breathe-ease® XL solution contains no preservatives.

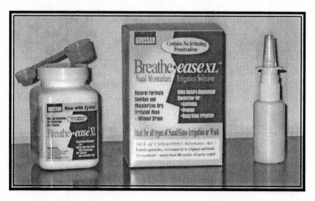

Figure 13. Breathe-ease® XL Irrigation Solution and Spray Bottle

I am certain other nasal sprays will continue to be developed that offer symptomatic relief of nasal and sinus issues. I have tried, for example, another nasal spray known as Xlear®, which is purified saline with xylitol and grapeseed extract. This spray is soothing and tastes mildly sweet, and it can be purchased at a local health food store.

Nasal Gels

Nasal gels also offer improvement of moisture content in the nose for all sinus, allergy, postnasal drip and ENS sufferers with longer-lasting effects than nasal sprays (which is helpful, particularly before bedtime). One criterion for nasal gels is they should be water soluble, meaning they can be dissolved in water; a gel that is not water soluble might cause harm to the lungs. One gel I have used is Breathe-ease® XL Nasal Moisturizing Gel, which can be applied directly inside my nostrils and then I gently close them to spread out the gel. This gel was originally developed for people who get sick when they fly. It provides moisture at the nasal and cellular level, which is ideal in the dry air of flight.

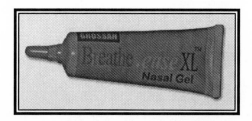

Figure 14. Breathe-ease® XL Nasal Moisturizing Gel

Another water soluble nasal gel, Ayr® Saline Nasal Gel, can also provide long-lasting moisture content without harmful preservatives, such as benzalkonium chloride. It comes in a tube and can often be found at a local pharmacy.

Nasal Oils

Nasal oils can be helpful in lubricating dry nasal passages for many hours while also preserving cilia functioning. They can also clear nasal passages and ease nasal congestion. Nasal oils are not a replacement for "washing out the sinuses" through irrigation or nasal sprays, but they do offer supplemental help.

Two common nasal oils are Ponaris® Nasal Emollient (which may be available at your local pharmacy) and Nozoil® Nasal Spray (which is available via the Internet). From my experience with these products, I have found Ponaris® to have a menthol aftertaste and it seems a bit messy. Conversely, Nozoil®, which is pure sesame oil, is a spray and it is generally clean.

One warning about nasal oils: it is important to keep in mind these sprays are oil, meaning they are *thick* or viscous. Products we place in our nose might eventually drain into our bronchial airways. Frequent, long-term use of such oils might contribute to problematic issues in these passageways, potentially leading to pneumonia. Be careful.

MEDICAL REMEDIES

Irrigation with Antibiotics

If used properly (correct dosage and duration), antibiotics are a safe, effective way to rid your body of bacterial infections and they can be administered in various ways including orally, intravenously, and topically. They might be necessary to treat an infection and can save lives. You must talk with your doctor who will guide you on the most appropriate antibiotic for your particular situation, as you would obviously not put antibiotics in irrigation without an infection or your doctor's orders.

As mentioned earlier, Dr. Davidson introduced the concept of putting antibiotics into saline irrigation solutions for treating an infection. I focused on this method of antibiotics because it consists of having the antibiotic come into direct contact with bacteria and it can avoid side effects of systemic antibiotics. As with any antibiotic you must follow your physician's directions and prescription.

Dr. Grossan's Guide for Adding Antibiotics to Irrigation

1. Add 1 teaspoon of salt to the Hydro Pulse® basin.
2. Add 500 cc of warm water and mix.
3. Make sure the stream is about 1 inch high.
4. Irrigate the nose 300 cc (about 150 cc each side) to thin the mucus.
5. Stop and gently clear the nose.

Then, after 300 cc has been used, do the following:

Add medication to the remaining 200 cc. This medication might consist of 40 mg of gentamycin® solution; tobramycin®, particularly for patients with cystic fibrosis; while others might use half a tube of bactroban®; and still others might use antifungals because of a link between rhinosinusitis and fungi.

1. Irrigate about 100 cc on each side until empty.
2. Sit quietly for 10 minutes at the sink. No blowing.
3. After that, sit quietly for 10 minutes to keep the solution in longer and do not blow the nose for two hours, so as not to blow medicine in the ears via the eustachian tubes.

Guaifenesin

Guaifenesin is a benign over-the-counter medication that has been helpful for thinning mucus in my nasal passages, so it might also be beneficial for sinus, allergy and postnasal drip sufferers. This medication is a mucolytic meaning it helps thin mucus by increasing the amount of water in mucus. It is unknown exactly how it works, although it is possible that it serves as a muscle relaxant, helping one to reduce stress and thereby thin mucus.[3] It is a systemic drug, and I have found that the brand Mucinex® extended-release (which comes in 600 mg tablets, with a maximum of 2400 mg per day) seems more effective than the generic brands of guaifenesin (which come in immediate-release tablets at a dosage of 400 mg), most likely because of the longevity of its effect.

Zinc Lozenges

Zinc lozenges are rich in antioxidants and help to improve resistance to infection so they should be helpful for sinus, allergy, postnasal drip and ENS sufferers. Some studies reveal that taking zinc lozenges at the start of a cold reduces both its severity and duration. I have found that to be true and I have also noticed that zinc lozenges coat my throat when it is irritated. However, high doses of zinc should be avoided because it can be toxic and suppress immune system function.

It is important to beware of nasal spray or swab forms of zinc. These products have been associated with anosmia and resulted in lawsuits in 2006.[4] When sprayed directly into the nose at relatively high concentrations the zinc can lead to burning and destruction of olfactory epithelium, the nerve cells responsible for smell. Some users have permanently lost their sense of smell as a result. Remember, if there is a chance for nasal irritation or damage, the ENS nose is more sensitive than a healthy one.

Allergy Shots

I highly recommend allergy shots (also known as immunotherapy) if you are experiencing allergies, whether or not you have ENS. As an ENS sufferer with allergic rhinitis, allergy shots are helpful for me in improving my nasal health and MCC functioning. I often look forward to them with anticipation.

After undergoing a series of tests from an allergist to determine which allergens trigger your allergic response (e.g., grass, pollen, dust, mold, animal dander), allergy shots are administered in increasingly concentrated doses over weekly, bi-weekly, tri-weekly and then monthly intervals. These shots are often administered for 3-5 years for optimal benefit. These shots offer long-lasting protection from allergies by reducing levels of IgE by producing another antibody known as blocking-IgG.

Allergy shots have been shown to decrease mucociliary transport time after one year of use, according to one study that included Dr. Houser as one of the researchers.[5] The transport time was determined by testing how long saccharin takes to travel throughout the nasal cavity.

Antihistamines

Antihistamines (allergy pills) can dry out the nose further but I believe, and it has been my experience, that antihistamines can be helpful if an ENS sufferer has allergies. Antihistamines work by blocking a histamine (a biochemical in immune system responses) from binding to a receptor site. That is, they prevent an allergic response from happening. I use lubricated eye drops to offset the effects of using an antihistamine daily, since antihistamines or drying agents in the nose can also contribute to dry eyes.

Three Vaccines

1. The pneumonia shot is helpful in reducing some of the bacteria in our lungs, and it should not be administered more than once every 5 years. It is a simple, protective factor that can certainly help sinus, allergy, postnasal drip and ENS sufferers fight infections.

2. The flu shot, given on a yearly basis (generally in the fall), is also helpful in fighting infections and preventing the flu. The flu is a respiratory illness caused by influenza viruses, and it can lead to, among other medical problems, pneumonia, sinus infections and ear infections.

3. The haemophilus influenzae type B (Hib) vaccine can also be beneficial for the ENS sufferer. Hib disease can cause pneumonia, inflammation of the throat, and in more extreme cases bacterial meningitis, which occurs when bacteria reach the spinal cord or brain. While children over 5 years old and adults usually do not need the Hib vaccine, it can be considered for those with "special health conditions" such as a weakened immune system, as is the case with some ENS sufferers.

Decongestants

Decongestants can dry the nose out further for ENS sufferers. Your doctor should guide your use of these drugs.

Oral decongestants cause blood vessels of the nose to shrink in size. Although they might be helpful during an upper respiratory infection such as a cold, one side effect I have noticed is they accelerate my heart rate. Consequently, they should be used cautiously if you have high blood pressure and their stimulant properties contraindicate long-term use due to potential adverse effects on the heart.

Anti-inflammatories

Anti-inflammatories reduce inflammation of nasal and sinus membranes. They can be beneficial if you are a sinus, allergy, postnasal drip or ENS sufferer since these conditions all exhibit inflammation. The use of corticosteroid sprays is one example of an anti-inflammatory medication that can be helpful and should not damage the nasal mucosa, particularly at low doses. Although they sometimes have preservatives such as benzalkonium chloride, they are only administered in low doses, usually once per day.

Various natural anti-inflammatories have been proposed to help reduce inflammation while not having a drying effect. Dr. Grossan recommends bromelain (pineapple enzymes) taken on an empty stomach to help thin mucus. Three studies from the 1960s, as well as one recent study, have found that bromelain is helpful in improving sinusitis symptoms.[6-9]

Quercetin with bromelain is another remedy I have found helpful. It is helpful for people with ENS and allergic rhinitis by reducing inflammation and supporting immune system functioning.

Other natural remedies include Colostrum®, flaxseed oil, Chlorella Growth Factor®, and nonsteroidal anti-inflammatory drugs (NSAIDS). These natural anti-inflammatories, however, represent alternative medicine and have not been evaluated by the Food and Drug Administration (FDA). They are generally allowed to be on the market if they do not make unsupported scientific claims. Please view the American Herbal Products Association (AHPA) website at *www.ahpa.org* for objective information on herbal products.

DIETARY REMEDIES

Plenty of Fluids

I believe water is one of the best drinks for anyone suffering from sinusitis, allergic rhinitis, postnasal drip, or ENS. Water is considered the universal solvent because it dissolves more substances than any other liquid. It is also a mucolytic since it helps thin mucus by increasing its water content. By making the mucus thinner, it drains better. People with sinus or chest infections often do not drink enough fluids and they could benefit greatly from drinking eight 8-ounce glasses of water per day to wash away toxins in their bodies and enjoy improved health. Warm water can be particularly helpful as its warmness can soothe the throat; conversely, ice cold water might "freeze" or slow down the cilia, and should be avoided.

In addition to water, other juices that offer sinus benefit include orange and dark grape juice. These juices not only have mucolytic properties, but they are also high in Vitamin C and can therefore bolster your immune system. However, parents take note: drinking too much juice might cause someone not to be hungry at dinner since these juices contain much sugar, leading him or her to miss out on other important nutrients.

As an ENS sufferer I bring two 12-ounce water bottles to work every day. If I do not drink at least 12 ounces of water (or another fluid) during the day, I incur significant postnasal drip and my voice becomes raspy. Drinking water has been very important for me in keeping mucus moving.

Hot Tea with Lemon and Honey

Dr. Grossan believes hot tea with lemon and honey is one of the best mucus thinners.[10] He recommends drinking 8 cups of tea a day when you have a cold or sinus condition, including postnasal drip.[11] Tea, black or green, contains a chemical compound called EGCG (epigallocatechin gallate), which blocks allergic responses and stimulates cilia action.

I have found hot, green tea particularly helpful and soothing, and it is also high in antioxidants. Some teas contain caffeine while others do not. It might be wise to avoid tea that contains caffeine in the evening so it does not keep you awake at night, interfering with your sleep cycle.

Chicken Soup

Chicken soup is another great natural remedy that is beneficial for sinus, allergy, postnasal drip and ENS sufferers because it helps thin mucus. Chicken contains an amino acid called cystein that is similar in composition to the drug acetylcysteine, which is used to treat respiratory problems, including bronchitis. The chicken in the soup can help thin mucus, which in turn makes the nasal and bronchial cilia move quickly, better defending the body against infection.

Vitamins (Particularly A and D)

Vitamins in general are a good, safe option for any sinus sufferer since the diets of Americans, who show rising rates of obesity, often lack proper nutrients. I take a multi-vitamin every day for good health. Other nasal conditions, such as atrophic rhinitis, have been associated with vitamin A deficiency; vitamins A and D are also helpful in producing mucus, which improves moisture content in a dry nose of someone with ENS.

Dietary Considerations

In general, green, leafy vegetables, fresh fruit, and foods high in protein are helpful for sinus, allergy, postnasal drip and ENS sufferers because of their nutritional value. Conversely, caffeinated products such as chocolate, coffee, or certain sodas might lead to increased dryness and should be avoided, particularly during the evening so they do not interfere with sleep.

Despite its tendency to make one drowsy, alcohol has been shown to have adverse effects on sleep cycles.

Smoking is discouraged because it might not only worsen the lungs, but it could also exacerbate the already present breathing difficulties with ENS.

Another dietary consideration for ENS sufferers is food allergies, which are much more common in children than adults and far less common than environmental allergies. Food allergens are proteins within food that are not properly broken down by heat when cooking or by stomach acids when digesting food. Because they are not broken down, they survive to move from the gastrointestinal lining to the bloodstream, then entering various organs, thereby causing an allergic reaction.

Shellfish, peanuts, fish and eggs are common food allergens for adults, while eggs, milk and peanuts cause more problems for children. Adults with an allergic reaction to food generally have to deal with them for life, while children sometimes outgrow them.

Products to Avoid

- Caffeinated products
  - Chocolate
  - Coffee
  - Certain sodas
- Alcohol
- Tobacco smoke

Foods that Promote Healthy Sinuses

◆ **Vegetables:** broccoli, lettuce, spinach, carrots, cauliflower, and potatoes. These vegetables are rich in nutrients and maintain their nutritional value if eaten raw or steamed.

◆ **Fresh fruits:** pineapples, bananas, apples, pears, oranges, grapes, and kiwi.

◆ **Spicy foods:** hot peppers. They clear your sinuses for the moment—if your stomach can handle it!

◆ **Wheat products:** rice, oatmeal. These foods help aid digestion. People with ENS are sometimes anxious, which can contribute to an irritable bowel.

◆ **Foods high in protein:** meat, milk, fish, and cheese. These foods are particularly beneficial during times of infection since they help repair tissues and cells and improve immune system functioning.

Environmental Remedies

Environmental Considerations

Mold and dust mites are two prevalent types of allergens that can be found everywhere, particularly in the home. Cleaning your home by frequently dusting, mopping, or doing laundry helps to improve the quality of the air you breathe, and has helped to improve my nasal breathing. The use of an air purifier or allergen-proof pillowcase can also help.

Humidifier

The use of a humidifier can also be helpful for people with ENS to increase moisture content in the air, which can help moisten nasal passages. A humidifier can offer significant benefit for all sinus, allergy and postnasal drip sufferers. It is dry during winter months in New York, which is why I use a humidifier primarily during that time of the year. Indoor humidity should be kept between 40-50%, a level that can be determined through purchase of a hygrometer. Humidity above a 50% level, however, can lead to the creation of mold spores and dust mites, which should be avoided. Since outdoor humidity is often above 50% during warm, moist times of the year, a humidifier would not be beneficial during that time.

Furthermore, it is important to follow the manufacturer's directions when cleaning a humidifier. Otherwise the humidifier can lead to an increase of bacteria and mold, and it will re-circulate them, which could do more harm than good. Fortunately, there are some humidifiers, such as an evaporative humidifier, that have built-in self-cleaning functions and do not require as much maintenance.

If you wish to humidify the air but do not wish to purchase a humidifier, you can simply pour water into shallow aluminum pans and the water will evaporate. Another relatively low maintenance way to humidify the air is a vaporizer, which works by boiling water and requires minimal cleaning.

Good Hygiene

This topic might seem self-explanatory but it cannot be overemphasized. As discussed earlier, rates of primary atrophic rhinitis are low in the Western world due in part to the use of antibiotics and improved oral hygiene. Clearly, hygiene plays a role in promotion of good health. Three basic activities that seem important for sinus, allergy, postnasal drip and ENS sufferers are brushing and flossing your teeth, taking a warm shower, and washing your hands.

Brushing and flossing your teeth prevents bacterial infections from setting in. Given the proximity between the nose and mouth you want to keep both of them free of bacteria. Some products that might be helpful are made by TheraBreath® and can be purchased at *www.therabreath.com.* These products include a specially-formulated toothpaste, an oral spray that dissolves tonsil stones (bacterial debris toward the back of the throat), and a Hydro Floss® machine to remove plaque buildup.

Taking a warm shower will also help because of the steam that is warm and humid. Sinus, allergy and postnasal drip sufferers will benefit from this moisture because it will keep the mucus moving, while ENS sufferers benefit from the moisturizing of their dry nasal passages.

Frequently washing your hands is also important because illness-causing bacteria and viruses can get onto your hands. Transfer of bacteria by touching your food, your face or your eyes with dirty hands can increase the likelihood of catching an illness. Obviously, that is not good for the sinus or ENS sufferer because of his or her already weakened immune system.

Principle 2: Maintain Blood Supply to the Nose By Stimulating Remaining Turbinate Tissue

Key Strategies

✦ Exercise

✦ Swimming

✦ Warm Packs

✦ Other methods:

    1. Acupuncture

    2. Biofeedback

    3. Inversion Techniques

Exercise

Regular exercise (perhaps 30 minutes a day, 3 days per week) can not only increase blood supply to remaining turbinates for ENS sufferers, but also provide protection against depression for all sinus sufferers. Stimulating blood flow to the brain while increasing levels of serotonin reuptake inhibitors will decrease the likelihood that someone will develop depression. Exercise, however, is difficult for ENS sufferers in cold weather because cold air irritates the nose and lungs. I would often note some throat and bronchial irritation after running outside in fairly cold weather, below 55°F. Running should be done in a well-ventilated area, perhaps at a local gym where the air is neither too hot nor too cold. Some ENS sufferers can indeed run long distances. I mentioned in chapter 3 that I ran a 9.3 mile road race in 2002 and 2006, and my family physician has asked if I would consider running a 26 mile marathon with him next year. That seems like quite a feat for an ENS sufferer, but I am confident it is possible with training and practice.

Swimming

I am not much of a swimmer, but I can understand why swimming might be helpful for someone with ENS. Not only does water offer increased moisture in the air, but also one reaps the benefits of exercise when swimming. It might be particularly helpful for an ENS sufferer who otherwise has difficulty engaging in vigorous exercise such as running. When swimming, I recommend using nasal plugs because pools usually have chlorine in them, which can irritate the nose when going underwater.

Warm Packs

I purchased a Sinus Bed Buddy® from a local Bed, Bath and Beyond store, which is a small blue bean bag that can be heated in a microwave. Applying warm packs to the sinuses can improve blood circulation for sinus and ENS sufferers. Warm, moist towels applied to the sinuses might similarly improve blood flow.

Other Methods

Below are 3 other methods that increase blood flow to the turbinates. Except for the inversion technique, I have not attempted the other 2. I include them in this book because some ENS sufferers have benefited from them.

1. *Acupuncture* consists of inserting fine, sterile needles throughout the body along "meridians," which might help alleviate some headache and facial pain for sinus and ENS sufferers. It is based upon an ancient Chinese belief that physical and mental health depend upon a natural flow of energy along the 14 pathways, known as meridians. This technique must be done by an acupuncturist as it would be dangerous to do by yourself.

2. *Biofeedback* has been helpful for ENS sufferers as it simply consists of providing information that tells the body what to do. Dr. Grossan suggested an example of biofeedback as follows: look in the mirror and watch your face relax. The more you see your face and jaw relax, the more likely you are doing it correctly because of the feedback you are receiving.[11] Through biofeedback an ENS sufferer can learn to relax and breathe more comfortably. One study, for instance, showed how asthmatics reduced their asthma severity from moderate to mild through biofeedback.[12]

3. *Inversion techniques* consist of keeping your head lower than the rest of your body to get more blood flow to the brain and upper body. One way to practice an inversion technique is by lying on your bed with your head facing downward off the side of the bed for a couple minutes. I would exercise caution not to apply too much pressure to your eyes, ears, or nose or to do it for too long (more than a few minutes) because a blood vessel could burst. People with ENS, including myself, who have tried this technique found it helps increase blood flow to the missing turbinates, offering nasal relief for a short time.

Principle 3: Relax

Key Strategies
✦ Sleep
✦ Reduce Stress

Sleep

Getting enough sleep each night has significant bearing on how my nasal health is the following day. It is suggested the average adult should get between 7-9 hours of sleep per night, with 8 ¼ hours about average. Sleep is the body's way of naturally healing and it aids in promoting good health for all sinus and ENS sufferers.

Because of sleep-disordered breathing in ENS, the use of a Continuous Positive Airway Pressure (CPAP) machine, with a built-in humidifier, might be helpful in improving the quality of sleep. A sleep specialist would need to prescribe it.

A second helpful idea for improving the quality of sleep is an electric, reclining bed. A bed that allows slight elevation of the upper body allows for easier breathing because of less pressure on your lungs than when you are on your back in what is called a supine position. While a pillow might allow for sufficient elevation for some, a reclining bed might be an improvement because there is no risk of getting a stiff neck.

Reduce Stress

We live in a high-stress society with many demands and expectations. Stress can play a negative role in anyone's nasal health by leading to increased sinus infections. I have found that my sinuses generally feel better and are less inflamed when I am relaxed, as opposed to when I am under much stress. While everyone relieves stress in different ways, participating in enjoyable activities, taking a vacation, playing a sport with a friend, and praying are examples of ways to reduce stress. The bottom line is whatever you find relaxing and enjoy doing can help you reduce stress.

Tips to Reduce Stress

- Do what you enjoy: listen to music, take a warm shower, or read a novel.
- Enjoy a massage, particularly if your muscles are tense. A massage has been shown to reduce pain, boost immunity, and decrease blood pressure.
- Pray. Even a few minutes of meditation either at the beginning or end of the day can be rejuvenating and good for your health.
- Find humor in the small things since humor has a way of diffusing negative emotions.
- Try to stay positive. Remember, negative feelings such as anger, anxiety and depression can consume you, while positive, optimistic thoughts can literally boost your immune system.

Chapter 9 References

1. Zitner, A. (2001, May 10). Sniffing at empty nose idea. *Los Angeles Times*, p. A.1.

2. Subiza, J. (1999). Inhibition of the seasonal Ige increase to dactylis glomerata by daily saline nasal - sinus irrigation during the grass pollen season. *Journal of Allergy and Clinical Immunology*, 101, 387.

3. MeSH Descriptor Data. Retrieved November 24, 2006, from the National Library of Medicine—Medical Subject Heading Web site: *www.nlm.nih.gov/cgi/mesh/2k/ MB_cgi?term=Guaiacol+glycerel+ether.*

4. Leaving you senseless? Retrieved February 11, 2007 from the ABC 15, KNXV TV, Phoenix Web site: *www.abc15.com/news/investigators/index_story.asp?did=33189.*

5. Cmejrek, R.C., Gutman, M.T., Torres, A.J., Keen, K.J., & Houser, S.M. (2005). The effect of injection immunotherapy on mucociliary clearance in allergic patients. *Otolaryngology- Head and Neck Surgery*, 133, 9-15.

6. Kataura, A. (1965). Treatment of chronic sinusitis by the combined use of protein-ase p-741 (bromelain) and antibiotic (erythrocin). *Jibiinkoka*, 37, 381-385.

7. Hine, S., & Tamura, N. (1966). Clinical use of bromelain (ananase) in chronic rhinosinusitis. *Jibiinkoka*, 38, 439-442.

8. Kagitomi, T., & Shozuka, K. (1966). Effect of bromelain in chronic sinusitis. *Jibiinkoka*, 38, 433-437.

9. Braun, J.M., Schneider, B., & Beuth, H.J. (2005). Therapeutic use, efficiency and safety of proteolytic pineapple enzyme Bromelain-POS in children with acute sinusitis in Germany. *In Vivo*, 19, 417-421.

10. Grossan, M. (personal communication, November 1, 2006).

11. Grossan, M. (2004). *How to be free of sinus disease – permanently!* Los Angeles, CA: Hydro Med.

12. Biofeedback helps asthmatics breathe easier. Retrieved April 8, 2007 from the Applied Psychophysiology and Biofeedback Web site: *www.aapb.org/i4a/pages/ index.cfm?pageid=3629.*

Chapter Ten

━━━━◦◦◦━━━━

Surgical Treatment Options

I f an ENS sufferer is experiencing breathing difficulties and he or she has not experienced sufficient improvement from the non-surgical techniques just discussed, then 2 surgical approaches, currently done by only a few doctors in the United States, may be performed. These surgical techniques focus on narrowing the nasal passageway by two means: by closing the nostrils (Young's procedure) or by implanting biomaterials under the mucous membrane. The latter technique is far more practical and the primary surgical option discussed in this chapter.

The first surgical technique, Young's procedure, consists of bilateral closing of the nostrils to prevent further atrophy of the nasal mucosa. This procedure should be done at 3 month intervals. It is difficult for me to imagine spending 3 months with my nostrils closed. More recently, a modification of this procedure has been to only partially close the nostril to allow for internal examination of the nose. Regardless of its apparent disadvantages, results from this operation include disappearance of nasal crusting six months after the procedure, and an increase in the length, but not number, of cilia.[1] Perhaps using nasal plugs (which help maintain moisture in the nose) long-term could produce a similar outcome, although it might be inconvenient wearing them due to their large size and tendency to fall out.

Various materials can be used to implant and thereby reconstruct the nose including bone, cartilage, muscle, and fat, as well as biomaterials such as plastipore, Goretex Dualmesh®, and Alloderm®. Implanting such materials seems far more practical and perhaps just as, if not more, effective than Young's procedure.

Submucous implantation of biomaterials to alleviate symptoms—breathing difficulties, nasal dryness, sleeping problems, and depression—associated with atrophic rhinitis and ENS has been practiced for over 100 years. Given the conservative nature of turbinate surgeries during the first half of the twentieth century, implant surgeries were then more often indicated for primary atrophic rhinitis. Because of the increasingly aggressive turbinate surgeries practiced and decreased incidence of primary atrophic rhinitis in the Western world during the second half of the twentieth century, such implant surgeries were more often indicated for either ENS or secondary atrophic rhinitis.

Wachsberger in 1934 considered implant surgery "unwarrantedly unpopular" because of 1) the unknown etiology of atrophic rhinitis, 2) the fear that these implants would lead to scarring, which made it difficult for a doctor to accept how they would help the patient, and 3) the lack of familiarity with standard surgical procedures for primary atrophic rhinitis.[2]

Gersuny in 1900 was the first doctor to do implants by injecting paraffin (wax) under the nasal mucosa.[3] Dr. Cottle used cartilage (from the septum, ears, or ribs) and cancellous bone for implantation of the nasal floor, lateral wall and septum in the 1950s, describing this technique as "exceptionally valuable" and highlighting the very positive effects implants had on his patients' nasal health and emotional well-being.[4] He recommended performing this technique every 10-20 months for 5-10 years to reach optimal nasal benefit.

While the idea behind these implants was to allow less air to enter the nose, resulting in less drying of the nasal mucosa and subsequent increase in mucosal secretions, Dr. Cottle offered a more elaborate explanation. In his 1958 landmark article "Nasal Atrophy, Atrophic Rhinitis, Ozena: Medical and Surgical Treatment," Dr. Cottle suggested some of the most important effects of these implants included increased nasal airflow resistance to enhance pulmonary functioning and nasal airflow that was more calm, orderly, and fast.[4] He reported that, through repeat surgeries, some of his patients became completely asymptomatic and demonstrated remarkable improvement to their mental health.

During recent years, a number of researchers have reported some relative success using implants. Rice reported success using hydroxyapatite cement on one patient; Goldenberg reported excellent results using plastipore on 6 (of 8) patients; and Friedman, Ibrahim, and Lee, along with Moore and Kern, indicated some success with Alloderm®.[5-8] Friedman et al. reported 5 (of 7) patients indicated significant improvement from Alloderm® implantation on their inferior turbinates, and Mendonca, Alves, Voegels, and Butugan reported all 12 patients experienced improvement of symptoms by implanting cartilage, bone and silicon on their inferior turbinates.[9] (However, Mendonca et al. did note that patients with an early stage of atrophic rhinitis reported more improvement than those with an advanced stage, known as ozena.) Wang, Liu, Qu, Dong, and Yang reported using ilium (bone of the pelvis) on 5 patients resulting in improvement of symptoms, while Papay, Eliachar, and Risica presented using muscle for implantation with similar improvement.[10-12]

Yet these researchers acknowledge they have only helped to alleviate the severity of symptoms, and most of them did not present a long-term follow-up on the stability of their results beyond a few years.

Dr. Houser uses Alloderm® because it is fibrous tissue that does not require the patient to donate his or her own body parts. Alloderm® has low absorption and rejection rates assuming that the proper technique of stimulating blood vessel growth into the implant is applied during surgery.[13] According to Dr. Houser, the Alloderm® implant initially shrinks about 10% immediately after implantation, just like what happens to a dry, folded tissue when it gets wet. But after blood vessels grow into it (a process he estimates takes at least 3 months from surgery), the size of the implant remains stable.

Cymetra®, on the other hand, is micronized bits of Alloderm® mixed with saline that can be injected, eventually turning into hard form. However, because the effect might be small as it spreads, it is very challenging to apply a large volume of Cymetra® on its own as an implant, but it can be used to increase the size of an already existing implant. In fact, several patients have reported benefit from topping off their Alloderm® implants with Cymetra®. Cymetra® is performed as an office procedure, so it is less costly than an operation, but its outcome seems rather minimal. It is nevertheless possible it might have a larger cumulative effect if it is repeated many times with long-time intervals between injections to allow proper incorporation of blood vessels and to ensure most of it does not turn into scar tissue. However, its stability on the size of implants over time has not been studied.

Finally, SIS® has been primarily used for septal perforations, but not for treating ENS. One of the difficulties in using SIS®, as Dr. Houser personally showed me, is that it is too thin and fragile, requiring numerous sheets to achieve a bulky implant. Consequently, Alloderm® is the preferred implant of choice for treating ENS.

Such implants help to improve nasal humidity, regulate heat, filter air, re-direct airflow, and restore normal nasal sensations. According to Dr. Houser, Alloderm® implants have been successfully implanted with his longest implanted patient (4.5 years after surgery) still presenting stable results.

An Alloderm® implant can be implanted underneath the submucosa anywhere in the nose—including the septum, nasal floor, lateral wall, and directly into the turbinate. It is placed into the submucoperiosteal or submucoperichondrial layer (which is the membrane that separates the nasal submucosal layer from the bone or cartilage, respectively), depending on whether it is the cartilagenous part of the anterior septum or the bony skeleton of the rest of the nose and septum.

Alloderm® is often implanted into the septum, opposite the sight of the missing turbinate tissue. The only place to implant to compensate for a removed middle turbinate, for example, is the septum, opposite the resected main body of the middle turbinate. Dr. Houser does not implant directly into a partially resected middle turbinate because it is a thin, delicate structure, making it hard to raise a flap and insert anything even if the turbinate is full in size. An implant into the septum, on the other hand, grossly but quite effectively mirrors the shape and size of the resected turbinate.

In some cases it is beneficial to implant the nasal floor, although usually done as a last resort, to increase nasal airflow resistance and direct airflow toward normal tissue and the olfactory bulbs, likely improving the patient's sense of smell. Use of the nasal floor also supplements an implant into the septum, as it allows the total size of the implants to be larger. People with ENS-IT might particularly benefit from implantation on the nasal floor because, as research has demonstrated, airflow tends to remain in the lower portions of the nose among those with ENS-IT.

Implanting the lateral wall in patients whose inferior turbinates are largely removed, right under the bone shelf of the resected turbinate, also remains a possibility. But the submucosal layer of that site is very thin and therefore difficult to handle. And since most inferior turbinate resections are in the anterior end of the turbinate, very close to the nasolacrimal duct, special care should be taken not to damage or block this duct. This is why the majority of researchers have not attempted to implant there. However, Mendoca et al. reported good results implanting there among patients with complaints of paradoxical nasal obstruction, and Dr. Houser believes it remains a good site to implant under the hands of a skilled surgeon. There is logic in not abandoning this site for implantation since the inferior turbinate naturally extends horizontally along the lateral wall.

If much of an inferior turbinate remains, at least 40%, then Dr. Houser recommends it can be augmented with Alloderm®. If less than 40% remains, he believes it will be more beneficial to implant one or more of the previously mentioned sites.

Dr. Houser has pioneered a method of implanting spear-shaped cuts of Alloderm® into a partially resected inferior turbinate, when at least 40% of it is remaining. The intent is to augment the remaining turbinate tissue with Alloderm® so that it gains more normal size and shape.

For further information and updates regarding implants, please visit Dr. Houser's website at *www.geocities.com/shouser.html*, where you can peruse an implant tutorial. Dr. Houser is presently conducting research on the effectiveness of Alloderm® implants among his patients, which includes my own results (you can check regularly for updates). Hopefully, as awareness continues to grow regarding the debilitating effects of ENS, more ENT doctors will develop interest in designing and implementing implants that can help rebuild missing turbinates.

Like everyone who suffers from a chronic disorder, ENS sufferers hope for a cure. Recently Dr. Stephen Badylak, a research professor in the Department of Surgery and director of the Center for Pre-Clinical Tissue Engineering at the McGowan Institute for Regenerative Medicine, used pig's bladder to regenerate a finger tip—with encouraging results![14] Within six weeks the bone, blood vessels, nerves, skin, and fingernail all grew back. ENS sufferers hope the same can happen for our turbinates. While this study is encouraging, we continue to cope by utilizing the best surgical remedy available, which is presently an Alloderm® implant.

Chapter 10 References

1. Young, A. (1971). Closure of the nostril in atrophic rhinitis. *Journal of Laryngology and Otology*, 81, 515-524.

2. Wachsberger, A (1934). New technic in surgical treatment of ozena. *Archives of Otolaryngology*, 19, 370-382.

3. Gersuny, R. (1900). Ueber eine subcatane pothese. *Ztschr.f.Heilk*, 1, 199-204.

4. Cottle, M.H. (1958). Nasal atrophy, atrophic rhinitis, ozeana. *Journal of the International College of Surgeons*, 29, 472-484. [P. 482].

5. Saunders, W.H. (1958). Atrophic rhinitis: results of surgical treatment. *Archives of Otolaryngology*, 68, 342-345.

6. Rice, D.H. (2000). Rebuilding the inferior turbinate with hydroxyapatite cement. *Ear, Nose, and Throat Journal*, 79, 276-277.

7. Goldenberg, D., Danino, J., Netzer, A., & Joachims, H.Z. (2000). Plastipore implants in the surgical treatment of atrophic rhinitis: Techniques and results. *Otolaryngology - Head and Neck Surgery*, 122, 794-797.

8. Goldenberg, D., Danino, J., Netzer, A., & Joachims, H.Z. (2000). Plastipore implants in the surgical treatment of atrophic rhinitis: Techniques and results. *Otolaryngology - Head and Neck Surgery*, 122, 794-797.

9. Moore, E.J., & Kern, E.B. (2001). Atrophic Rhinitis: A review of 242 cases. *American Journal of Rhinology*, 15, 355-361.

10. Mendonca, M.L., Alves, R.B.F., Voegels, R.L., Sennes, L.U., & Butugan, O. (1998, August.) *Atrophic Rhinitis: Surgical Treatment and Results*. Paper presented at the meeting of the XVII European Rhinology Society and International Symposium on Infection and Allergy of the Nose. Viena, Austria.

11. Wang, Y., Liu, T. Qu, Y., Dong, Z., & Yang, Z. (2001). Empty nose syndrome.

Zhonghua Er Bi Yan Hou Ke Za Zhi, 36, 203-205.

12. Papay, F.A., Eliachar, I., & Risica, R. (1991). Fibromuscular temporalis graft implantation for rhinitis sicca. *Ear, Nose and Throat Journal*, 70, 381-384.

13. Sclafani, A.P., Romo, T.III, Jacono, A.A., McCormick, S.A., Cocker, R., Parker, A. (2000). Evaluation of acellular dermal graft (AlloDerm) sheet for soft tissue augmentation: a 1-year follow-up of clinical observations and histological findings. *Archives of Facial and Plastic Surgery*, 2, 130-D.

14. *Make like a salamander*. Retrieved February 17, 2007 from the University of Pittsburgh School of Medicine Web site at: *www.pittmed.health.pitt.edu/Fall_2006/salamander.pdf*.

Chapter Eleven

Concluding Thoughts

Against my best wishes, I do not anticipate ENS becoming extinct in the current generation. I am relatively young (age 27 as of this writing) and I hope to be alive for a long time. However, as an ENS sufferer I have learned to cope and my situation has improved. Various management techniques and Alloderm® implant surgeries have been beneficial. I am unsure how much functioning of my nose I will recover and I do not anticipate a cure in the near future. In the meantime, however, I can do what is best to help my situation and continue to learn from others who are in a similar predicament.

ENS does not have to be an issue in the modern world. It is a surgery-induced problem that can be prevented in the future through ENT specialists and plastic surgeons implementing improved, conservative surgical techniques when operating on turbinates. It is my hope that ENT doctors will continue to develop and explore possible surgical remedies for reconstructing the noses of existing ENS sufferers; and that ENS sufferers, at the same time, can use various treatment strategies discussed to help them cope and share with one another what has worked for them through this book and websites such as *www.emptynosesyndrome.org*. I also hope that sinus, allergy and postnasal drip sufferers can use information in this book and resources in the appendices of this book to not only learn how to prevent or treat their symptoms, but also to learn some valuable lessons from ENS sufferers (not only what happens when a nasal surgery goes awry, but also treatment strategies that might prevent the need for turbinate surgery in the first place).

Overcoming ENS is not an easy feat by any stretch of the imagination. ENS is difficult to manage and it is hard to cope with. Lack of knowledge on part of doctors regarding this condition compounds the stress for the ENS sufferer. Hopefully, through publications such as Dr. Houser's research article "Empty Nose Syndrome Associated with Middle Turbinate Resection," through effective use of the empty nose syndrome website, and through patient testimonials, there will be increased awareness of ENS.

Raising awareness through heightened visibility of ENS is key in promoting treatments. Increased awareness will help ENS sufferers in the following ways including, but not limited to:

1. ENT doctors and plastic surgeons will become increasingly cognizant of this problem as to employ turbinate reduction procedures that will decrease the volume of the nasal airways, while making absolutely certain to preserve nasal mucosa. With greater caution taken by these doctors in general the incidence of ENS, whatever it might be, could decrease (or diminish entirely) in the future.

2. ENS sufferers will learn how to help themselves. An understanding of treatments that work for ENS, why ENS sufferers experience what we do, and an understanding of what surgical reconstruction options are available are all means to improve our individual situations.

3. By sharing stories with others and increasing understanding among others, ENS sufferers promote treatments for ENS. One way to do that is by sharing our symptoms with ENT doctors or plastic surgeons. One such symptom is feeling short of breath. If these doctors encounter the same problem repeatedly, they will

understand it is a real problem and should be taken seriously. Hopefully that is already happening. ENS sufferers can also advocate for themselves by sharing their stories with others, including friends, family, and even the media (via television or a letter to the editor of their local newspaper). The plight of ENS must be heard loud and clear, never to be forgotten lest the same mistakes are repeated in the future.

Finally, I implore you to show appreciation to doctors who are working to improve the condition of ENS and to promote awareness of this problem. Drs. Houser, Grossan, Tichenor, and Kern, to name a few, are some doctors to whom we already owe tremendous thanks. I am certain other ENT doctors and plastic surgeons more local to you, the reader, might also be working to promote the ENS cause and should be shown appreciation.

Joining as a united front, ENS sufferers, ENT doctors, plastic surgeons, research scientists, families, and friends can fight together on behalf of ENS. We ENS sufferers can become healthy, productive citizens, rather than increasingly paralyzed by this difficult-to-manage condition. Hope is on the horizon and help is on the way. We just have to search for and find it. God bless.

Appendix A

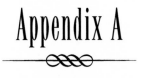

Glossary

Acupuncture: An ancient practice that uses sterile needles, inserted in strategic places, to help reduce pain.

Allergen: Substance such as pollen, dust or mold that causes an allergy.

Allergic rhinitis: When allergens in the air cause an immune system response consisting of production of immunoglobin E (IgE), in turn leading to inflammation of the nasal membranes.

Alloderm®: Dermal tissue stripped of all cells that is taken from a cadaver and is used as a biomaterial implant for empty nose syndrome.

Antibiotics: Medication that kills bacteria.

Antihistamine: An allergy pill that works by blocking a histamine from binding to a receptor site.

Anti-inflammatory: A drug that reduces inflammation of the mucous membranes.

Anxiety: Nervousness.

Aprosexia nasalis: A term used to describe difficulty concentrating.

Asthma: Reversible constriction of the airways, which become inflamed and lined with excessive amounts of mucus.

Atrophic rhinitis: An advanced state of empty nose syndrome that has resulted in mucosal atrophy and is often accompanied by fetor, which is a foul-smelling odor from the nose.

Biofeedback: Receipt of feedback regarding your body's functions, which can be helpful in improving relaxation and stimulating the body's natural defense.

Bromelain: Pineapple enzymes that can help improve sinusitis symptoms.

Caldwell-luc: Also known as traditional sinus surgery, a surgical tool where the maxillary sinus is entered above the gums.

Cilia: Millions of tiny hairs that help move the mucus blanket along by beating at a rapid rate—healthy cilia beat at 16 pulses per second.

Cotton: Use of saline-moistened cotton can be used to increase nasal airflow resistance and temporarily decrease ENS symptoms.

CPAP: Abbreviation for continuous positive airway pressure, often used by patients who have sleep apnea. A CPAP with built-in humidifier might be used by an ENS patient.

Crust: Dried mucus.

Cryosurgery: Freezing turbinate tissue to reduce its size.

CT scan: Three-dimensional images of a body using x-rays. An example is a CT scan of the sinuses.

Cymetra®: Micronized bits of Alloderm® that can be used as an injection to increase the size of an existing implant.

Decongestant: Medication that helps reduce congestion by causing blood vessels to constrict.

Depression: A pervasive feeling of sadness, sometimes brought on by learned helplessness or the perceived inability to control life's circumstances.

Electrocautery: Use of an electric current to heat tissue and reduce turbinate size, which is similar to radiofrequency.

Empty nose syndrome (ENS): A complication of nasal surgery that results from removal of too much turbinate tissue.

Endorphin: A natural, biochemical compound that kills pain and enhances emotional well-being.

ENS-Both: The subtype of ENS when part or all of the inferior and middle turbinates are removed.

ENS-IT: The subtype of ENS when part or all of the inferior turbinates are removed.

ENS-MT: The subtype of ENS when part or all of the middle turbinates are removed.

ENT doctor: A physician who specializes in treating problems of the ear, nose and throat, some of whom also perform surgery. They are also known as otolaryngologists.

Ethmoid sinuses: The pair of small sinus cavities that are between the eyes.

Eustachian tube: A tube that connects the middle ear with the pharynx.

Functional endoscopic sinus surgery: Operation in which an endoscope is used to examine and cut areas within the sinuses.

Gastroesophageal reflux disease (GERD): When acid in the stomach flows upward rather than downward.

Guaifenesin: A medication that helps thin mucus.

Histamine: A biochemical in immune system responses.

Iatrogenic: Directly caused by medical treatment. ENS is an iatrogenic condition because it is a complication of surgery.

Immunotherapy: Also known as allergy shots, immunotherapy is a course of progressively increasing doses of the shots to make the immune system less reactive to allergens. This has been shown to improve the mucociliary clearance system.

Infection: The result of when bacteria, viruses, molds, or fungi infect bodily tissues.

Inferior turbinate: The large turbinate that helps direct airflow while also having strong contracting and expanding capabilities. Given its size and location in the nose, the inferior turbinate is most often the obstructing turbinate.

Injection corticosteroids: A surgical injection to decrease the size of the turbinates.

Inversion technique: Keeping one's head lower than the rest of the body to bring more blood flow to the turbinates, which should be done very cautiously.

Laminar: When turbinates are present, air enters the nose in an orderly manner.

Larynx: The voicebox.

Laser surgery: Use of a laser beam to shrink or burn tissue.

Lavage: To clean or rinse.

Maxillary sinuses: The pair of large sinus cavities located under the eyes and behind the cheekbone.

Microdebrider: A hollow tube with a blade at one end and suction device at the other, which is often used during turbinate reduction surgeries.

Middle turbinate: The turbinate that is higher up in the nasal cavity, between the eyes.

Mucolytic: An agent that breaks down or thins mucus by increasing the water content in mucus.

Mucociliary clearance system: The process by which cilia sweep the mucus blanket that carries infectious particles to be harmlessly deposited in the pharynx. It is very important for fighting infections and overall healthy functioning of the nose.

Mucous membrane: Tissues that are rich in glands that have significant mucus-producing capabilities and line the nose, sinuses, respiratory and digestive tracts. It is referred to as mucosa for short.

Mucus: A substance that increases moisture within the nose and provides surface area to catch infectious particles. Mucus consists of 2 layers: the sol (thin) and gel (thick) layer above it. The gel layer traps particles and the entire mucus blanket—sol, gel, and particles—is transported per cilia to the pharynx where it is swallowed.

Nasal gel: A substance that can be applied to the inside of the nostrils to improve moisture content in the nose.

Nasal irrigation: Rinsing the nose and sinuses with salt water.

Nasal mucosa: Short for mucous membrane and it can be considered the organ of the nose.

Nasal oil: A viscous substance, such as sesame oil, that can lubricate the nose and sinuses.

Nasal spray: A spray to moisturize the nose and thin mucus.

Nasolacrimal duct: The drainage system that passively drains tears from the medial eye to the inferior meatus.

Olfactory epithelium: The mucosal layer of nerve cells responsible for detecting smell.

Olfactory nerves: Nerves that detect smell.

Otolaryngologist: Same as an ENT doctor.

Outfracture: A relatively safe procedure consisting of breaking a turbinate bone, and then applying pressure to move it toward the lateral wall or side of the nose.

Paradoxical obstruction: A confusing symptom experienced by ENS sufferers, which is a sensation of not being able to breathe adequately, stuffiness or partial suffocation, despite a wide open nasal cavity.

Parasympathetic nervous system: The autonomic nervous system that relaxes the body. This system slows the heart rate, increases intestinal and gland activity, and relaxes muscles in the digestive tract.

Partial turbinectomy: Reduction of the turbinates by about two-thirds.

Pharynx: The throat.

Phlegm: Thick, sticky, stringy mucus.

Plastic surgeon: A doctor who specializes in surgically changing the appearance and function of a person's body. Just like ENTs, they can reduce and remove turbinates.

Postnasal drip: A term used to denote thick mucus that has collected in the back of the nose and upper throat.

Pulsatile irrigation: Nasal and throat irrigation that pulsates. The pulsating action in nasal irrigation stimulates cilia to their natural rhythm, while throat irrigation increases circulation to the throat area.

Radiofrequency: A turbinate reduction surgery that uses heating to induce submucosal tissue destruction.

Rhinitis: Inflammation of the nasal mucosa.

Rhinorrhea: A severe runny nose.

Saline irrigation: Same as nasal irrigation.

Scar tissue: Non-functional tissue that has grown back over a wounded area.

Septal perforation: A hole in the septum, which is the midline of the nose.

Septoplasty: Surgery to straighten the septum.

Sinuses: Hollow cavities of the skull and face, consisting of four symmetrical pairs (maxillary, ethmoid, sphenoid, and frontal sinuses).

Sinusitis: Inflammation of the sinus membranes.

SIS®: Thin biomaterial from a pig that can be used for certain implants, but it is too thin for an implant for ENS.

Sleep apnea: To stop breathing during sleep.

Stress: The body's change or reaction to life activities. Two types of stress are distress (bad stress) and eustress (good stress).

Submucous resection: Turbinate reduction procedure that either removes part of the inferior turbinate bone or vascular space tissue underneath the mucous membrane.

Superior turbinate: The small turbinate high up in the nasal cavity and well out of the main airway that houses olfactory nerves. A superior turbinate is rarely touched during turbinate surgeries.

Total turbinectomy: A surgery in which entire inferior turbinates are removed, though stubs usually remain.

Turbinate surgery: Any surgery that involves reducing the size of turbinates.

Turbinates: Complex bony structures, which are covered by mucous membranes, that, among other functions, help direct, warm, humidify and filter air. They play critical roles in conditioning air as it enters the nose and consist of inferior, middle, superior and sometimes supreme.

Turbinectomy: A surgery in which part or all of the turbinates is removed.

Turbulent: Air enters the nostrils in a disorderly (too slow and haphazard) fashion due to the removal of the inferior and/or middle turbinates.

Vaccine: Medication given to boost immunity against an infectious disease.

Vasomotor Rhinitis: Primary symptom is a runny nose. The nerves of the nose that increase secretions are very active, resulting in a steady stream of thin mucus.

Water soluble: Can be dissolved in water.

Wheezing: Coarse, whistling sound produced in airways during breathing.

Young's procedure: A proposed surgical treatment for ENS that involves closure of the nostril(s) for 3 months to regenerate nasal tissue.

Appendix B

Websites of Interest

www.emptynosesyndrome.org

The empty nose syndrome website helps ENS sufferers connect with and support each other. It contains a lively discussion forum, a section where Dr. Houser answers questions, and a tutorial on both the nose and turbinates. A half-hour audio tape of Dr. Kern's lecture on empty nose syndrome is also available. David Lemberg of Nantucket, Massachusetts, is the owner and operator of this website. He is also co-founder of the Empty Nose Syndrome Association and patient support forum.

www.geocities.com/shouser144/index.html

Dr. Houser's website contains information on a variety of topics including, but not limited to, sinusitis, allergies, nasal and sinus surgery, and empty nose syndrome. Of particular interest is a tutorial explaining the Alloderm® implant procedure.

www.ent-consult.com

Dr. Grossan's ENT website features a forum where topics are discussed, including saline irrigation and sinus, ear and throat problems. Part of this website also includes a section of FAQs on sinus topics. Dr. Grossan directly answers questions from sinus sufferers by emailing him at *ENTconsult@aol.com*. Dr. Grossan also has an article on empty nose syndrome, which the site reports to have "received the largest amount of email of any of its web pages."

www.sinuses.com

Dr. Tichenor's website has won numerous awards for outstanding content. His website offers a variety of information on symptoms and treatments for sinusitis. There is also a section that includes other sinus diseases and new technologies for treating them. Empty nose syndrome is discussed in the post-surgery section of the website at *www.sinuses. com/postsurg.htm*. You might read his research paper, which is an attempt to encourage allergists to recognize postoperative complications, including ENS, at: *www.aaaai.org/media/resources/academy_statements/ practice_papers/endoscopy.pdf*.

www.pubmed.gov

The above website is a service of the National Library of Medicine and National Institutes of Health. It includes more than 16 million citations, some of which are from MEDLINE and other life science journals. Some of the articles are full-text.

www.mayoclinic.com

This website is a service of the Mayo Clinic, which is reported to be the first and largest not-for-profit group medical practice that seeks to treat every complex illness. This website offers numerous tools on various health topics. Of interest to the ENS sufferer is an explanation regarding saline irrigation.

www.webmd.com

This website is considered a leading online provider of health information to consumers, physicians, healthcare professionals, and employees.

Appendix C

Dr. Houser's Replies to FAQs

The following are the most frequent ENS questions asked of Dr. Houser, which were submitted onto the *www.emptynosesyndrome.org* website. Dr. Houser answered all of these questions. This is a compiled list of questions from patients and Dr. Houser's answers retrieved from the website on May 18, 2007.

Tests for ENS

What is a "cotton test"?

The cotton test consists of placing moistened cotton, or cosmetic puff portion(s), into the nose to see if inhibiting the airflow improves the symptoms. Symptomatic improvement suggests that an implant at that location would be beneficial. The implant likely increases nasal airflow resistance, directs air in an orderly fashion to the mucosa for sensation, while it also deflects air into an area that has maintained more normal sensation, one that is not operated upon, or has healed properly.

Do CT scans correlate with ENS symptoms?

A CT scan shows an overview of nasal and sinus anatomy and demonstrates if resection has taken place. It can also show infections and tumors, but it cannot be the only guide to turbinate work because symptoms are so important. There is no ideal nasal mold that all noses should resemble.

Is the saccharin test a good indicator of ENS symptoms?

The saccharin test measures mucociliary clearance. It is reasonable to think it will be down in a dry, ENS patient. The problem is that scar tissue from surgery can impede ciliary flow as well. That said, a prolonged saccharin time does not say ENS is the cause. Conversely, a quick saccharin time may mean the patient moisturized well that morning.

Alloderm®, Cymetra®, and Surgery for ENS

Does Alloderm® shrink over time?

Alloderm® when implanted usually has to be larger than the desired size—an overcorrection, as it "shrinks" a bit as the body incorporates the tissue. Imagine folding a piece of tissue paper 20x—seems fairly thick, now wet it—it "thins down" similar to the folded Alloderm® becoming incorporated. Basically all the air spaces and folds soften and go away as the body takes the implant over. Once it is incorporated I see it stay—longest is 4.5 years. Does it fluctuate early on while healing? Yes, absolutely, as the swelling from surgery comes and goes. Lifecell Corporation reports it will shrink in mobile areas, such as the lips; the nose is static. The nose does not have the stress in the lips. Once the implant is incorporated, it stays the same size for years. The longest follow-up for this surgery that I am aware of is 10 years out from Dr. Dean Toriumi: he placed Alloderm® on a patient's dorsum during rhinoplasty, and went back 10 years later for a revision; the Alloderm® was still present and viable.

Have you ever witnessed Alloderm® shrink in size and why might that be?

Of all the implant surgeries done, I have only witnessed one patient's Alloderm® shrink. A patient implanted 4.5 years ago for ENS-MT has had neuropathic pain and I have tried to cover his trigger site with submucosal Alloderm® with modest success. His pain began to come back so he returned.

The most recent implant, which consisted of a broad one placed at the posterior floor 8 months ago, seems reduced in size although it was enormous 3 months ago. Yet the Alloderm® that was placed 4.5 years ago in the septum remains fully in place and good-sized. It has NOT shrunk over these years. Here is my professional opinion on why that might be (please note this is just a theory without yet solid evidence supporting it): while the posterior nose has good blood supply, the graft was to a submucoperiosteal tunnel with little bleeding. The bone itself does not bleed much, and the tunnel does not much either unless disrupted. When I graft to the septum, the area has invariably been operated upon so I struggle to "find the plane" and am certainly out of the submucoperiosteal or submucoperichondrial plane. This transgression allows ingrowth of vessels. An untouched area with a "proper" plane can lead to poor vessel ingrowth and atrophy of the graft. From now on I will strive to disrupt the bony cortex (use of a curette, an instrument that can scrape tissue and get some bony bleeding) as well as the submucoperiosteal tunnel (pull some out from inside the flap). I do not think it was infection without symptoms, but that is still a possibility as well. Therefore, the reason Alloderm® may have shrunk is because it was placed into a bloodless plane, and this situation may explain why some doctors claim Alloderm® resorbs. Crafting a blood-rich field becomes the solution.

How long does it take Alloderm® to incorporate into the body?
I give patients at least 2 weeks of antibiotics post-implant to allow the area to remain sterile while healing is beginning to occur. Alloderm® is a foreign body until the body grows into it, so it is a race between bacteria and the patient's body. It then takes months for the body to fully incorporate Alloderm®. Based upon clinical experience, Alloderm® will become incorporated in 6 weeks for a small graft to 3 months for a large graft. I would need to do animal studies to give you a more exact answer than that.

Where is Alloderm® implanted?

This depends on where tissue is missing from. It is placed either submucosally into the inferior turbinate, or subperichondrial to the septum, or subperiosteal at necessary bony locations. Seeing a CT scan gives me an idea where tissue is missing and what can be done, but physical exam and scoping are ultimately of greater importance. Is the lateral wall no good per Dr. Michael Friedman? Yes, the lateral wall without inferior turbinates is tough to graft. I implant the inferior turbinate if it is of adequate size, otherwise I resort to the septum. Lateral wall grafts are limited by the nasolacrimal duct inhibiting a large graft in the exact spot where it is most likely to help—near the head of the inferior turbinate. The septum will accept a graft below the lining and fill a similar space to the adjacent turbinates, or at least where they used to be.

**Why is Alloderm® implanted under general
rather than local anesthesia?**

Some can be done under local, but I prefer to do larger, posterior grafts under general anesthesia. Exact positioning of a graft requires the patient to be still. Going deep into the nose is more straightforward in a still patient as well. Bleeding in an awake, but sedated patient is dangerous. Doctors used to do most sinus surgery under local anesthesia as it was felt pressure on the dura would be noted and the doctor would stop the procedure. Anesthesia has improved, as well as surgical expertise, so general is now the preferred route.

Can the nasal cycle occur with implanted Alloderm®, or is this nasal function damaged?

Alloderm® will, over time, take on the characteristics of the tissue it is implanted into. If it is placed submucosally into the vascular capacitance tissue, then I believe it can take on this function partially. It will also form simple scar, fibrous tissue that is non-functional, but bulky. I do not believe the function is damaged, as radiofrequency or cautery treatmants to the submucosal tissue, which are more damaging to the submucosa than a tunnel or incision, are temporary. It does appear that some mild ability of the nasal cycle occurs in grafts. Grafts certainly become viable as they bleed readily when incised.

What about injectable Alloderm® (Cymetra®)?

It can work below a strong barrier such as perichondrium, periosteum, or Alloderm®. Cymetra®, when mixed at the manufacturers specifications, will burst the turbinate membrane. When mixed thinner it is less apt to do so, but it also spreads out farther, which equals less effect from the injection. I think Cymetra® stays, but you have to understand that the actual volume of Alloderm® injected in the form of Cymetra® is very small. Cymetra® has been disappointing as it is either too thick resulting in rupture and no enlargement so all falls out, or too thin, which ends up as a diffuse deposit. Perhaps the diffuse deposit over time might bring some relief, but how many injections are needed? Under a graft seems somewhat better as the Cymetra® can be thicker as it pushes against the Alloderm® above it, that then pushes against the mucosa above that. The solid graft allows the force to be distributed, so less chance of rupture. I believe that Cymetra® stays, but I cannot state with any certainty; as it spreads out it becomes tough to see in the nose as there is no visible bulge to watch or follow.

Can SIS® be used?

Sure, it is a collagen product, but porcine. It is thin, so many layers would be needed. Tissue clay? I am not sure. Silicon? It is a foreign body and tends to extrude or become infected.

How much does implant surgery cost?

This varies based on where and what surgical approach is used. Often the bill would be in the $5,000-15,000 range. I do not have control over costs, just CPT codes. I can do surgery on indigent patients from Cuyahoga City, Ohio, but others end up having to pay or use insurance. I have had pretty good luck getting coverage approved for patients.

Is the nose more moist after an implant?

This appears to be the case. As the rate of airflow is reduced, less moisture is stripped from the nose, hence the nose is more moist. Moisturization still remains important after the implant, though.

Can a turbinate be transplanted?

Not with current medical technology. The blood vessels deep inside the nose cannot be attached. Nor would immunosuppressives be wise or accepted here. Can mucosa be grafted? There are no donor sites from the same person. The nose has respiratory epithelium; the answer is no.

Would it be possible to rebuild at least the turbinate bone on top of the resected turbinate?

A bone substitute can be placed there. See Dr. Dale Rice's article for an example. A thin shelf of bone is tough, and it is not a small undertaking. It would consist of a lengthy healing, it would require frequent cleaning sessions, and it may fail.

Once respiratory epithelium, which includes cilia, has gone through metaplasia, can it be revived? Can too much moisture or humidity be bad to the mucosa or cilia in any way?

Yes, the cilia can recover if the offending cause is removed and normal tissue—not scar tissue—surrounds it. The cilia are meant to be "underwater" as the pericilliary fluid, or sol layer, surrounds them and the entire nasal epithelium. Isotonic saline should not damage cilia.

Treatment Thoughts

What is your take on the use of cotton to improve symptoms?

While I know patients who use cotton on a regular basis with no aspiration or problems, medico-legally I cannot tell someone to use this technique. You should discuss this technique with your ENT or primary doctor before attempting it, and perhaps your ENT will place the cotton. What I advise patients is to tie a thread to the cotton before placement and to tape the string to the nose or face. This will keep the cotton from being aspirated and allow for easy removal. Only use it for a few hours at a time as it will collect secretions. Is there still risk? Yes, as the thread can break, so it should be attempted with great care. It is dangerous to leave cotton in at night, because of the risk of aspiration. I have had patients experiment with cotton placed per tweezers and figure out where I need to put an implant. ENS-IT (or possibly ENS-Both) patients can often give good feedback. ENS-MT is too hard for a patient to get it to the right spot. I think a Q-tip is a good idea, as it is easy to withdraw, firm and too large to aspirate. Further, do not stick anything straight up into the top of the nasal vault as the skull is thin up there and injury could result. Use your head and be careful.

Are vitamins helpful?

Vitamins are wise for everyone as our diets tend to be poor. I am not aware of any vitamin or homeopathic remedy for ENS, but neither am I aware of any that will worsen the condition.

Can't growth factors induce growth or hypertrophy of the remaining tissue?

Vascular endothelial growth factor (VEGF) and similar compounds can induce vascular proliferation in the heart. These medicines risk blindness through vessel ingrowth at the retina, but this risk is offset by revascularizing an ischemic area within the heart. ENS is severely debilitating, I agree, but one could argue not life-threatening. The nose is so close to the eye that I would suspect the eye would be a great risk from an intraturbinal injection of a growth factor. Certainly blindness has been reported from intratur-binal steroid injections. I doubt the FDA would ever approve VEGF for intranasal injection.

Patient Experiences

While most ENS patients have most of the front of their turbinates cut, have you examined ENS patients with the opposite problem of having most of the front turbinates but little of their rear turbinates?

I do recall one patient with ENS who was missing the back of the left inferior turbinate. A cotton test to the area brought significant relief.

Have you seen patients who are missing their turbinates but not reporting symptoms?

Yes, I have seen multiple patients who are missing turbinates, middle or in-ferior, but never both yet, who are completely asymptomatic. They might be seeing me for sleep apnea or an ear issue. I am always a bit surprised and I will push them about their breathing, trying to elicit some ENS symptoms, but none are reported.

Have you had a patient whose turbinate symmetry is perfect but they experience different symptoms in each nostril?

A patient of mine had 3 turbinate surgeries and, after a turbinate surgery in August 2006, he is left with 25% of the inferior turbinates bilaterally and 80% of the middle turbinates. It is too early to know if his ENS symptoms will persist—still some time to possibly resolve; I saw a woman resolve by approximately 10 months after surgery. The fascinating issue is that he has ENS symptoms on the right but NOT on the left, yet his anatomy is absolutely symmetric. Cotton test on the right brought notable symptom improvement, but no change on the "normal" left side. Now we have living proof that ENS is more than just turbinate resection, but another "domino" must fall as well.

I want to sue the doctor who did my surgery. Will you help?

I cannot help in this area. I am trying to gather ENS patient cases to research and publish this information. Being an expert witness helps an individual, but would discredit the work I am trying to accomplish, which may help many patients.

Is there any circumstance in which ENS might seem less severe than the problem before surgery?

In France, a procedure is done termed nasalization—a euphemistic term. It is a fairly radical, aggressive approach to remove turbinates and strip mucosa. But it is performed only on patients who have severe, refractory, obstructive nasal polyps. Perhaps these patients do get some ENS but when they compare their sensation to that prior to surgery, they actually feel better.

Other Thoughts

Are other doctors working on ENS?

The others that I am aware of are: Dr. Michael Friedman in Chicago, Dr. David Slavit in New York City, and Dr. Dale Rice in Los Angeles. There may be others. Those listed are variably interested, but there may be a starting point closer to home.

What do you believe is the incidence of ENS?

We may never know the true incidence of ENS. Hopefully as awareness builds then the standard of care will be NOT to remove turbinates, with no more ENS-IT, ENS-MT, and ENS-Both.

What is your stance on turbinate reduction procedures?

I believe turbinate reduction can be done safely per outfracture, radiofrequency, cautery, and submucosal resection. Even these conservative means can give a bad result though if overdone—too much energy is delivered. I do not think laser treatment serves much use, as destroying mucosa to get at the target tissue is unwise. I am not fond of partial turbinate excision. Decongestion and a skilled operator can get around the turbinate in such cases. The risk of ENS is too great to do this for nasal obstruction. I do not believe total or near-total turbinate excision is correct unless cancer is suspected, or a severe problem exists and optimal visualization or exposure is needed, as in the case of a cerebral spinal fluid leak (CSF).

Why cannot medicine solve this through tissue engineering?

This may be possible in the future, but not at this point in history. A turbinate contains multiple components and it hangs suspended in space within the nose. A narrow attachment makes establishing blood supply to a graft a difficult or even impossible prospect. Vessel anastamosis is not possible deep in the nose, as it requires open visualization such as in the neck. Yes, cartilage and cartilage structures can be grown, but a turbinate also needs to have a covering of respiratory epithelium and submucosa below. Respiratory epithelium cannot reliably be grown at this time.

Appendix D

Books of Interest

Bruce, D.F., & Grossan, M. (2007). *The Sinus Cure: 7 Simple Steps to Relieve Sinusitis and other Ear, Nose, and Throat Conditions.* New York: Ballantine Books.

Grossan, M. (2004). *How to be Free of Sinus Disease—Permanently!* Los Angeles: Hydro Med.

Hirsch, A.R. (2004) *What Your Doctor May Not Tell You About Sinusitis: Relieve Your Symptoms and Identify the Real Source of Your Pain.* New York: Warner Books

Ivker, R. (2000) *Sinus Survival: A Self-help Guide.* New York: Penguin Putnam, Inc.

Josephson, J. (2006). *Sinus Relief Now: The Ground-breaking 5-step Program for Sinus, Allergy, & Asthma.* New York: Perigee Trade.

Kennedy, D.W. & Olsen, M. (2004). *Living with Chronic Sinusitis: A Patient's Guide to Sinusitis, Nasal Allergies, Polyps, & their Treatment Options.* Long Island City: Hatherleigh Press.

Metson, R., & Mardon, S. (2005). *The Harvard Medical Guide to Healing Your Sinuses.* New York: McGraw-Hill.

Timmons, B.H. & Ley, R., Eds. (1994). *Behavioral and Psychological Approaches to Breathing Disorders*. New York: Plenum Press.

Williams, M.L. (1998). *The Sinusitis Help Book: A Comprehensive Guide to a Common Problem: Questions, Answers, Options*. New York: John Wiley & Sons, Inc.

Appendix E

Index

About the Author

A fter developing empty nose syndrome as a result of surgery in 1997, Chris completed 7 years of college and is a nationally certified school psychologist in Upstate New York.

Despite living with empty nose syndrome for the past 10 years and knowing how tough it can be, Chris still considers himself tremendously blessed because he is married to his beautiful wife Colleen, has two sweet daughters, Faith, age three, Abigail, age one, and an unborn baby on the way.

Below is a photo taken in November 2006 of Colleen (top left), Chris (top right), Abigail (bottom left), and Faith (bottom right):

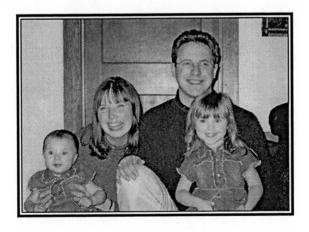

Please visit Chris' blog at *emptynosesyndrome.blogspot.com* to give feedback or ask questions about the book.

CPSIA information can be obtained at www.ICGtesting.com
Printed in the USA
LVOW080753090113

314971LV00001B/126/P